FD 2.0

A FLEXIBLE NUTRITION PHILOSOPHY FOR THE MODERN ATHLETE

BY KRISSY MAE CAGNEY

FD 2.0

A FLEXIBLE NUTRITION PHILOSOPHY FOR THE MODERN ATHLETE

BY KRISSY MAE CAGNEY
EDITED BY DREW CANAVERO
DESIGN BY RYAN COX

TABLE OF CONTENTS

A Note From the Designer

Since coming aboard, I've always played a supporting role in Krissy's professional world. I'm of course honored to call her one of my most treasured friends. It's been about a year since we first published Flexible Dieting, a project we knew we wanted to do even before relocating across the country. When we wrote it, edited it, designed it, we had little idea that it would have the impact that it has had. We are very proud of it, and we are thankful and humbled by the people we have helped, even if it's just in some small way. It made the long nights with little sleep and the passionate arguments about how to say what she wanted to say completely worth it.

In the time since, after reading thousands of emails and seeing hundreds of clients going through dramatic life-altering changes, there are a few insights I've gained that I feel compelled to share. When it comes to diet, like most things in life:

There is no single path.

All the information we present- all the mathematics, all the science, all the verifiable hypotheses- act as signposts towards a greater understanding of how you and your body work. These signposts form a roadmap. Like any map, when followed properly, will lead you to the place you want to be. Just like navigating the world, there are different routes and different paces you can take to reach your goal. But if you follow it, you will arrive. And just like you can't blame a map for not following directions, the same goes for your nutrition. The most someone else can do for you and your nutrition is to show you the signs and highlight the routes. It is up to you to follow them.

More importantly, a question has grown in the back of my mind: Does Flexible Dieting need an alibi? That is to say: does Flexible Dieting need a built-in excuse or a defense to justify its existence or to make it credible?

The simplification of Flexible Dieting into memes of pizza and ice cream with passionate captions attacking straw man critics with, "I eat this and I am still seeing results!" isn't the right approach for us. Not anymore. We are beyond that.

There is no need to justify Flexible Dieting on those terms. The only argument Flexible Dieting needs is its results.

The memes do approach and obliquely (albeit somewhat ineffectively) address the biggest challenge for Flexible Dieting: confronting the language of nutrition and the fundamental premise that foods are inherently good or bad, healthy or unhealthy, and shifting the conversation from food itself to peoples' relationships with food.

The idea of foods being "good" or "bad" or "healthy" or "unhealthy" is pervasive. It permeates the language of health and nutrition and therefore peoples' understanding of both. There is no singular or universal definition of what makes a food "healthy" as opposed to "unhealthy".

This concept becomes further confused when individual foods are conflated with the totality of foods consumed by an individual. A diet of pizza is different than a diet that includes pizza. Looking at a single food a person consumes isn't the same as looking at all the foods a person consumes. You can eat "unhealthy" foods and still have a "good" diet. That is one of the central tenants of flexible dieting.

All of this confusion of course makes for prime marketing opportunities. With diets, most arguments about "good" or "bad", "healthy" or "unhealthy" are tautological: A Fad Diet, or a Diet With a Fancy Name will start with a feeble and sometimes esoteric theoretical or philosophical premise. Then it will build a series of criteria that define "health" and "nutrition" in a way that ultimately supports the Diet With a Fancy Name's assertions and recommendations. "Diet With a Fancy Name works!" say the people affiliated with Diet With a Fancy Name, because it fulfills its own criteria.

Flexible Dieting isn't a diet. It is the assessment of the caloric needs of an individual and partitioning those calories into an appropriate range of macronutrients in order to realize the individual's goals by optimizing the body for improving body composition and performance and generally improve medically recognized markers of health. Diets end. But eating is the one thing you will do besides breathing you will do for the rest of your life. How long can you really go without a bite of cake, or a candy bar, or a doughnut, a piece of pizza, an ice cream cone, a bowl of cereal? More importantly, why would you want to resist in perpetuity? To what end? Why would you want to develop orthorexia or a generally unhealthy relationship with food? Food is supposed to make you survive and thrive and bring you joyous experiences. Food can only kill you if you let it. Flexible Dieting is a way to eat for life that allows for living. So go out there and live.

Ryan Cox

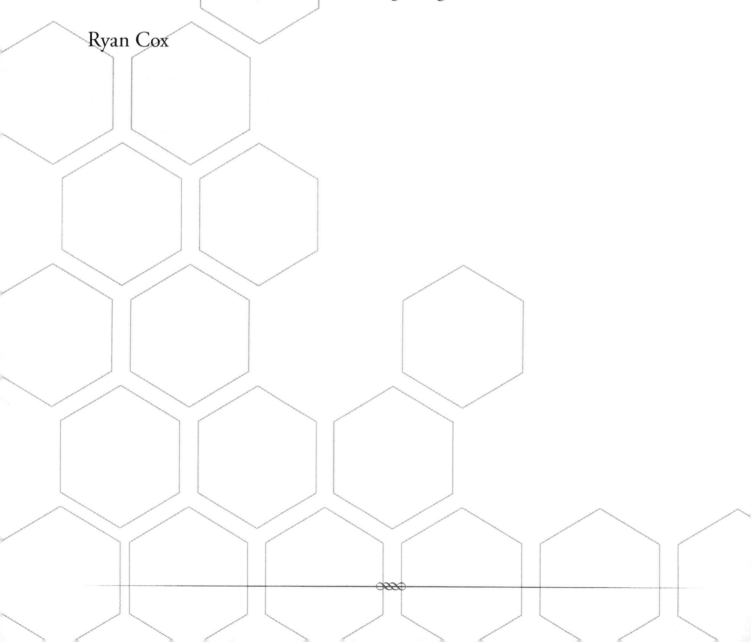

A Note From the Editor

This book was an idea long before Krissy started writing it, and enlisted my help to edit. And like most good ideas, it took a long time to gestate, to mature, and become what it is today. The book, in that respect, mirrors the evolution of its author. Flexible Dieting 2.0 stands not only as an addition to, but in some ways, a departure from, the ideas presented by its predecessor. The content, for the most part, is the same. The science and principles underpinning flexible dieting are unchanged (though more complete). What has changed-and will be immediately apparent to those who have read the first book-is the character of the person delivering that content. With respect to her candor, assertiveness, and yes, sarcasm, she is still the same woman we know and love. But she is more humble, more self-effacing, and more cognizant of the fact that, to remain a highly sought after voice in this industry, she must remain, for reasons beyond her sex appeal and sailor's mouth, a voice worth listening to. And in this book, Krissy has found her voice. The tenor of her mission—to improve people's lives through the practice of flexible dieting—and the passion with which she pursues that goal is no less steadfast, even as her tone has softened. Conciliation should not be confused with contrition; it is not to make amends for anything that Krissy has sought to clarify, and in some instances correct, statements and positions that, in the past, she was often intractable. Intractability drives wedges between people who would otherwise be friends and collaborators, and creates divisions where common ground could otherwise be built. These days, Krissy is anything but intractable. She has become more flexible in every respect, including her diet, and has reaped the benefits, personally, professionally, and competitively. She is one of those rare people who, in spite of the often retrograde forces of success, has learned to better follow her own advice. She's no longer just someone worth listening to; she's someone worth emulating. An example worth following, and a story worth telling. I'm honored that I get to play some part in helping her tell that story.

Drew Canavero

Foreword

If you have ever attended one of my nutrition seminars, you've heard the first question I ask: "Who has heard of 'If It Fits Your Macros?'", at which point I immediately rejoin, "Flexible Dieting is not IIFYM". I think I did an alright job in my first book explaining that one can't get by on eating calorically dense junk food, but I was far from thorough, or emphatic enough, about that point.

The first edition of Flexible Dieting was released in February of 2014, without the expectation that it would be so widely read. There is a lot of information available to read online when it comes to flexible dieting and I didn't expect to stand out from the crowd in any way. I specifically wrote it for my clientele in hopes to reduce email volume by compiling information into a short ebook that could answer the questions I was receiving. It was a very entry level, novice text designed to explain the basics for people who had never heard of flexible dieting. It helped a lot of people get started and that is something I'm proud of. The first book was designed to improve people's mindset when it comes to food, and teach moderation.

If I am being honest, I didn't reread my own book too often in 2014.

I started getting emails from very active individuals and I realized how many people were needing a 14 multiplier. I found myself giving people 15 multipliers, then having to explain why a 15 wasn't in the book. Once I had the attention of a few professional athletes, I needed to make 16 an option, as well. (You will see that the new book has an improved, more detailed multiplier scale).

I reread my book in September of 2014 and said two things to myself:

What am I trying to prove with my writing style? I was slightly abrasive and immature in the first book, and it was obvious that I felt like I needed to defend flexible dieting and justify my eating behavior. When I reread the book, it sounded like a sales pitch to me and that's not what it was intended to be. I want my writing to be well researched and a learning tool for whomever is reading it. So I started doing research daily to better support my claims and explain my message as opposed to me being an asshole and suggesting people listen "just because". I want my products to be well regarded and to be of the highest quality. This meant interviews, sources, better design, and an editor.

This is not suitable for athletes. The information was a great starting point and only that. There wasn't anything specifically written for an athlete as I only touched the surface of many important subjects rather than delving deep. I wanted to present something that could benefit every athlete.

The second realization made me notice that there isn't much out there with regard flexible dieting for athletes. It also made me realize I wanted to create something that would change the way people view themselves. The end goal is to get more people to actually envision themselves as athletes rather than just people trying to lose weight.

This is when I made the decision to do a full rewrite to better suit an expanding and increasingly diverse audience. Which brings me to the tile: "FD 2.0: A Flexible Nutrition Philosophy for the Modern Athlete". Who is the modern athlete? You are, whether it's your first month using a barbell or you're an Olympian. There are obviously different scales of athleticism, and even if you are at the very bottom of that scale with 100 pounds to lose, you are still an athlete if you are training hard and you should treat yourself accordingly. Your body is no less valuable even if, unlike a professional athlete, your body isn't your livelihood.

Another thing worth mentioning is that I toyed with the idea of renaming the book "Flexible Nutrition" as the word "dieting" has somewhat of a negative connotation. However I refrained for two reasons, (1) familiarity purposes, and (2) I don't want anyone to think that I am attempting to reinvent the wheel, hence the tagline "a flexible nutrition philosophy", as that's precisely what it is.

Before you start reading, be forewarned about some major changes you will see. Unlike the first book, there are no rigid rules in place, there's no requirement that you hit your macros dead-on, and there are more options this time around to help you achieve success. Enjoy!

1. Intro

I do not know where you currently stand with your fitness and nutrition journey. You may be a weight room veteran or you may have just signed up for your first gym membership yesterday. Whether you run marathons, powerlift, bodybuild, cross-train, play a professional sport, or take group exercise classes, we all have the following in common:

1. We all need to properly and adequately fuel our active lifestyles through intelligent and effective nutrition practices.

2. Most of us want to look good naked and desire a body fat percentage well below "average".

3. We all like to feel energetic, strong, and healthy.

There are several ways to achieve all of these objectives at once; however, after 10 years in the fitness industry, thousands of clients, a handful of competitions, a number of internships, and hundreds of hours of reading research studies, I've come to believe that there is one method of nutrition that truly trumps all others. That method is flexible dieting.

There are a few different definitions of flexible dieting, and I want to immediately clear something up: flexible dieting is not the same as a dietary free-for-all where you are encouraged to eat anything "if it fits your macros". IIFYM is a trend that is essentially a very misconstrued form of flexible dieting. People take it way too literally, and because of this unfortunate misrepresentation, there is a common misconception that flexible dieters live solely on junk food. We will discuss this further in Chapter 3. Being flexible with your eating does not mean you get to eat like an 8-year-old for the rest of your days. And while I don't believe in depriving ourselves of the food we love, nobody can live on doughnuts alone, and eating too many (even if they fit your macros) will result in some negative side effects. Armi Legge has provided a pretty solid notion of what flexible dieting truly is:

> *"Flexible dieting is about eating a diet you can maintain and enjoy, while keeping the body you want. Flexible dieting is not about counting calories or macronutrients. It's not about eating tons of junk food and hoping for the best. It's about finding the simplest, most effective ways to get the body you want with as little effort and anxiety as possible."*

I agree with Armi's definition because I think that being truly free of dietary restraints whilst remaining lean, strong, and healthy is ultimately everyone's goal. It takes a very long time, and a lot of legwork, to learn how to live this way. The most successful way for most people to achieve true nutritional flexibility is through educating themselves on calorie balance and macronutrients (not just learning how to count and track them). This is a process, as it goes far beyond simply knowing what protein, carbs, and fats are. You must become a self-examined athlete and you must be consistent and patient in the learning process. You need to treat your individual journey as a research study that may last for several years. Dieting is very unique to the individual and if you are going to retain any piece of information, you must always remember that your goals, level of activity, and palette are exclusive. Flexible dieting is about being flexible with yourself, not about imitating other people's eating habits who diet flexibly. It is no secret that I consume a fair amount of doughnuts, however most people don't have my training schedule, thus a superfluous feeding of pastries will not work for everyone. Here is my definition of flexible dieting:

> *"Flexible Dieting is the scientific approach to nutrition by finding a system that works for you in order to achieve your current physical and training goals. True flexible dieters shouldn't live by any set of rigid rules but by a relaxed set of flexible guidelines. This is a lifestyle and it needs to be treated as such. Try not to think of flexible dieting as a counting and tracking system, but as a simple and effective way to reach your goals with minimal angst and maximal potential. All while consuming the foods you love."*

There still is no consensus definition for flexible dieting, but that is the beauty of it. Flexible dieters agree upon the general guidelines, then apply them independently to suit their needs. You create your own rules from the fundamentals, you take responsibility for your nutrition, and you empower yourself.

The point of this book is to educate you and help you become a healthier, happier, and more athletic version of your current self. I have compiled my own knowledge of flexible dieting as well as provided you with information from some very intelligent people who have been pioneers in the nutrition field over the last few years. There will be a list of research studies at the end that you can read in order to further educate yourself, as my writing is simply to provide you with the rudimentary framework (and a little bit more) of this approach. If you are a competitive athlete, you may want to do further research in order to optimize your diet.

Wrapping your head around nutrition can be extremely difficult, largely because of conflicting information that is readily available in abundance all over the Internet. The amount of information—or, more aptly, misinformation—out there is completely mind blowing. Everyone has an opinion, and you can't be sure where people are getting their information. The worst place to soak up nutrition knowledge is in the squat rack or over coffee with a neurotic friend who has a history of fad dieting. The best places to find credible information are classrooms, nutrition seminars conducted by qualified individuals, research studies, and pertinent up-to-date reading material. The issue is that many can't afford the first two options and many may not be able to interpret the second two. So consider this my best attempt yet to give you the necessary information from all of the above.

Why you should rethink your dieting habits…

Nutrition is the single most important aspect of everything we work toward in our training lives, and when our diets are not on point, our training efforts seem to be for naught. It is no secret that how you eat determines how you look, feel, and perform. We all want to look great, we all want to feel amazing, and we all want to perform well. Enter the two most common dilemmas we see in nutrition, especially with athletes; the first being the bigger concern for women and the second being the bigger concern for men:

I need to eat less if I want to lose weight but I need to eat more if I want to perform better. This isn't always the case and later in the book, I will explain why. There is a particular way to manipulate your macros that allows for the athlete to become leaner without strength or performance suffering much, if at all. Weight loss is a result of tissue loss and tissue can mean fat or muscle. The goal with a person who is trying to lose weight is do everything possible to ensure most of that weight is fat loss. In order to maximize weight loss results, especially for an athlete, it is necessary to determine an effective macronutrient breakdown designed for performance and leanness. I do think one goal should take precedence and one should be secondary, but as progress is made, goals can be changed accordingly.

I need to gain weight in order to move a heavier barbell load but I don't want to lose my definition. We know it takes weight to move weight. The bigger a person is, the stronger they usually are—assuming we are talking about someone who is athletic. Gaining weight does not have to mean gaining fat. Of course tissue growth typically means both fat and muscle growth, but with flexible dieting knowledge of macronutrients, you can minimize the development of fat and maximize the development of muscle.

By now you know that in order to lose weight, specifically body fat, one must achieve a negative caloric balance by eating at a deficit and/ or intensifying training and activity. Conversely, in order to gain weight, specifically muscle, one must achieve a positive caloric balance by eating at a surplus and/or adding volume and minimizing conditioning and cardio.

Underpinning the efforts in both cases is a common refrain: be smart about it. Being educated on nutrition will give you results that are comparatively quicker, and more permanent. When leaning out, the end goal is to eat as much as you can whilst still dropping bodyfat. When making #gainz, you want to be consuming just the right amount to promote muscular growth but not consume so much that your body stores excess calories as fat. There is really only one smart way to do these things without driving yourself completely insane: remove all guesswork by determining your ideal caloric and macronutrient intake and adjust accordingly. Doing this is precise, efficient, and operative. It is also a method based strictly on science.

The next assumption that many people make when they want to lean out is that dieting isn't fun, which couldn't be further from the truth. Most people "diet" and go to extremes by completely omitting their favorite foods. Why are you punishing yourself for wanting to become a better version of yourself? I can't emphasize the following two statements enough:

1. *If you resent your training and are completely miserable, you need to do something else if you want it to go anywhere.*
2. *If you resent your eating habits and are completely miserable, you need to do something else if you want it to go anywhere.*

This text will hopefully open your eyes to better ways to eat, how to eat your favorite foods guilt free in moderation, how to maximize muscular development, how to maximize fat loss, and educate you on how to make all of these things permanent features of your diet, regardless of your goals. If the concept is new to you, it may be difficult to wrap your head around at first, but please keep an open mind while reading and absorbing this. You may have a hard time accepting the fact that you can be lean, strong, and eat ice cream everyday. You don't want to believe this because of how much nonsense the health and fitness industry has hammered into the minds of consumers over the years (the fat loss industry is a $60 BILLION a year industry that wants your money), but it can be done. I will teach you, and explain how it's possible through flexible dieting.

Do you have to manipulate and track macronutrients in order to get lean? Not at all. You can eat at a large caloric deficit and get lean fairly quickly via starvation. However, not only will you be miserable and hungry, but taking the expedient route will guarantee that you will lose the results just as quickly as you got them. If you train intensely, you need to eat the part. Eating enough at a caloric deficit is the trick.

Do you have to track macros in order to get big and strong? Not at all. You can eat at a large caloric surplus and get big and strong. However, if you are not tracking and monitoring your intake, you will likely add just as much fat as muscle (if not more). Gaining weight can be just as hard as losing it and eating everything in sight is far from an optimal, intelligent approach. You will also probably feel like a slow, lethargic piece of garbage.

People and athletes have obviously been getting results for years without flexible dieting, but things have changed. There has been a recent movement in the industry as we wanted to be bigger, leaner, faster, and stronger. We are willing to do whatever it takes. The amount of research that has taken place over the past few years has shown us a lot and real science (not bro science) is the MVP in fitness nutrition now. The "eat less, eat better" method simply doesn't cut it anymore because we have evolved. We are hungry for more, literally and figuratively speaking.

This book will provide the tools needed to determine what your body needs in order to reach your goals, whatever they may be. You can quit worrying about whether you ate too little or too much. You can give up feeling guilty about having a doughnut (or three) because everything is allowed in moderation and no foods are off limits. Being able to manage your own diet and macros is an invaluable skill that you will have in your back pocket. It is liberating, as you will now be able to be independent as far as nutrition is concerned. You do not need a coach, dietitian, or nutritionist to hold your hand forever . It takes trial and error, but it's crucial that you become familiar with and attuned to your body so that you know exactly how much of what it needs in order to look, feel, and perform at its very best.

This text will be your guide to an evidence-based, organized approach on how to intelligently design your diet to improve body composition and improve performance. One must learn to see food as human gasoline and know how to make appropriate food choices that are goal specific.

First Of All: The Notion of "Clean Eating" Needs to Dissipate...

"Clean eating" is an ambiguous term. Clean means what the dieter wants it to mean and there is no precise definition for what the term "clean eating" actually encompasses. There is no list of "clean" foods and there is no list of "unclean" foods. The definition is unique to the eater, thus making the term "clean eating" a very slippery slope and the cause of many arguments. What one person considers clean may not be considered clean by another because there is (and likely never will be) no broadly-accepted definition of what constitutes "clean" or "unclean".

To better illustrate this artificial dichotomy, let's compare a bodybuilder with someone who eats a paleo-oriented diet. Brown rice is generally paleo-prohibited but is a "clean" staple in the bodybuilding world. Someone who eats paleo typically eats a lot of bacon and this is seen as a healthy source of fat and protein, however, many clean-eating bodybuilders wouldn't even think about eating bacon because of its high fat content. Dairy is off limits for those on a strict paleo diet, but Greek yogurt is a "clean" source of protein in the bodybuilding world. Peanuts are not paleo-approved, but other varieties of nuts are (granted, peanuts are technically a legume), and most fitness enthusiasts consider all-natural peanut butter "clean". Do you see what I am getting at? If we asked 100 random people for a list of "clean" foods, not one of those lists would be identical. They would have the very obviously "clean" staples of chicken, fish, and vegetables, but that would likely be where the similarities ended. As we moved further down each respective list, toward the margins, we could expect the disagreement to escalate.

Since there is absolutely no way to objectively define clean eating, there is no way to measure what effect this type of "diet" will have on an individual's lifestyle, overall health, or performance. This, of course, means there is no credible way to quantitatively compare the efficacy of so-called "clean" diets to other, less clean diets. Furthermore, people forget that not everyone is attempting to lose weight. Someone who needs to gain weight for any number of reasons needs to consume calorically dense foods that are often considered "unclean" if gaining weight is a struggle. Some people need to eat a lot more than others, and high-calorie foods can make that an easier (and more enjoyable) process.

Someone has most certainly told you that certain foods are "bad", and if consumed, will hinder your progress. Of course an abundance of processed foods can have a negative effect on your health and body composition, but I think what people truly fail to realize is that an abundance of any foods can have a negative effect on your body composition. If you eat 6,000 calories a day of protein shakes and doughnuts, you are going to gain weight. If you eat

6,000 calories a day of eggs and broccoli, you are going to gain weight (fat and muscle if you are active). Obviously, the latter would not have the negative impact on your health that the former would, but the weight gain would be inevitable if your body requires only 3000 calories a day to fuel your lifestyle and maintain your weight. Over-consumption of excess calories carries the risk of adverse consequences, regardless of which foods those calories come from, and if they are regarded as "clean" or not.

The first thing that you need to do is completely get rid of the notion that there are "good" and "bad" foods. Looking at any food as "bad" is not only unscientific, but it's extremely unhealthy and oftentimes counterproductive. From here on out we are going to start looking at food differently, and apply this new mindset to body composition and human performance. Take a more scientific approach and begin looking at food based on its macronutrient content, as opposed to looking at food as normatively "good" or "bad". When you see bacon, you see protein and fat. When you see Greek yogurt, you see protein and carbs. When you see a doughnut, you see carbs and fat, and so on.

Furthermore, we must be able to put every food in the following categories:

Nutrient Dense or Non-Nutrient Dense. Food rich in nutrients, primarily micronutrients, are what we call "nutrient dense" foods. These, of course, are going to be the foods we know are rich in vitamins and minerals. Things like fruits and vegetable are usually the first things that come to mind. Foods rich in iron, potassium, magnesium, calcium, and omega-3s are also what we would consider nutrient dense. Non-nutrient dense foods are what we typically consider to be less beneficial to our health, such as cookies, ice cream, pizza, fried foods, which can be sub-categorized into all of our favorite things, ever.

Calorically Dense or Non-Calorically Dense. Foods that are calorically dense have more calories by volume than foods that don't. There is a common misconception that calorically dense foods are "bad" but foods like nuts, avocado, and salmon are high-calorie, yet usually considered health foods. A lot of fruits, especially those with higher carbohydrate content, would also belong to this category of calorically and nutrient dense foods. Then there are foods like green vegetables, which are extremely nutrient dense while being calorically less dense (which is exactly why they are encouraged, especially while dieting).

Combining the above information will allow you to determine what is "healthy" or "unhealthy". It depends on who is eating what. "Health" varies from person to person and we all have different histories, goals, and lifestyles. If you are allotted less than 2000 calories a day, you will need a majority of your food to be nutrient dense and non-calorically dense. If you are allotted over 2500 calories a day, you have some more wiggle-room to eat calorically dense foods that are less nutrient dense (if you so choose).

What constitutes a "healthy meal" is just as ambiguous as "clean eating".

This is where you really need to use your brain. Many people would say that a cheeseburger and fries is an "unhealthy meal", but how do they figure? There is value in red meat (iron), a potato has a rich micronutrient profile, and lettuce/tomato/onion are all nutrient dense and non-calorically dense. Just because you add cheese, a bun, and you fry the potato, it does not mean that the health benefits disappear, you simply just added some extra carbs and fats. This is why you will see people eat an open-faced burger, as carbs are not the enemy, but some people need to consume less of them than others.

Overeating anything can cause health problems, and of course we are more likely to overeat things like doughnuts and french fries. They are delicious. But just because you can overeat something, does not mean that you inevitably will, or have to. Moderation and balance is key. No foods need to directly be avoided at all costs unless you have a medical illness that has been diagnosed by a physician (remember that your holistic wellness coach is not a physician. If they use crystals for anything other than decor in their office, they aren't qualified to diagnose you).

We will go into detail about what and when you, as an individual, need to eat based on your size, lifestyle, and goals. What is healthy for someone who is a 230 pound athlete may not be healthy for someone who is 130 pounds and fairly sedentary. More importantly, I believe that we need to individually define what healthy means and the definition must be contingent on current goals.

Rather than labeling food by someone else's standard of healthy, I hope you are able to begin to look at food by its macronutrient profile, nutrient density, and caloric density by the time you have absorbed this text. The best way to learn, is to read nutrition labels regularly and cultivate awareness.

> *"Flexible eating encourages us to look at the physiological value of food - the macro and micronutrient profile - as well as to determine whether or not it could potentially aggravate an existing health problem (whether diagnosed or undiagnosed). In other words: if a food doesn't hurt, it's not off-limits."* -Eat To Perform

Why strict meal plans suck…

Eating disorders run rampant in men and women, young and old, especially in the health and fitness industry. I want to engrain in you a healthy relationship with food. One of the unhealthiest practices in this industry that literally drives people insane is the "meal plan", and I have found that strict meal plans are one of the biggest culprits of ED.

The meal plan usually consists of 6 small meals a day with 7 almonds in between a few of those meals. Your portions are predetermined for you and you know exactly what to eat and how much of it. You look at said meal plan and know that you are going to have to prep a ton of food in order to stick to it. So you spend all day Sunday prepping, measuring, and organizing your Tupperware. You are exhausted before starting, but you are ready.

Tuesday hits and you forget two of your prepped meals in your refrigerator. Panic strikes. So you choose to starve all day and shovel in two Tupperware containers of reheated food when you get home because you don't know what other options you have. You are sickened with worry because you were told that your meals need to be evenly spread out in order to "speed your metabolism" but the day is ruined. You end up eating your feelings… at least those aren't premeasured into Tupperware. You have become an inflexible, yo-yo dieter.

What constitutes an inflexible dieter? One who eats against their personal preference to the point that is does more harm than good on both a mental and physical level. It is good to have self-control and moderation, but not to the point of extreme deprivation.

Keep in mind that something that can't bend will break. Especially your diet.

You don't have to eat reheated food from a Tupperware container 6 times a day to get lean or strong. You shouldn't live a life where you feel as though you are a slave to food. You should never experience feelings of guilt after eating. You need to eat for both physical and mental health. I want to teach you how to eat for life as opposed to eating for abs, a wedding, a birthday, a high school reunion, etc.

When you get put on a meal plan by your trainer/coach, unqualified friends, or even worse, by yourself after an afternoon spent googling, you are taking a very short-term approach. You can't be on a rigid meal plan forever; in fact most people can't even do it for three weeks.

When you fall off the meal plan, it's difficult to get back on. I know first hand. You have a doughnut, hate yourself for it, call the meal plan quits for the day, and binge. You promise yourself that you'll adhere to the plan tomorrow. This isn't the case with flexible dieting. If you have a doughnut, you track it, the macros in that doughnut get subtracted from your daily intake, and you carry on with your day. A little 250 calorie "whoops" won't kill your vibe, whereas a 2500 calorie binge on a dozen doughnuts will literally destroy a week's progress. You can adjust your intake with a 250 calorie hiccup; not so much with a 2500 calorie binge.

The battle is everywhere, all over the Internet and on the social networks. There is a heated debate between the flexible dieters and Tupperware tilapia people. I was once a Tupperware tilapia person. I openly admit it. I was brainwashed into thinking that structured meal plans were the only way to successfully stay on track. I thought there were "good" foods and "bad" foods. The bad foods were anything that wasn't on the meal plan. Some people really like structured meal plans because you receive a list of foods, you don't have to think, and you don't have to understand the science of anything. You cook, you eat, you repeat. Uncompromising, automated eating. This is the problem. For most people, there is absolutely nothing tenable about following a meal plan like this.

People on strict meal plans usually feel bound to them and even the slightest hiccup will produce a massive anxiety attack and overwhelming feelings of failure. If you want to enjoy your life and briefly step away from your rigid plan, you typically can't do it without crying yourself to sleep after. I know people who avoid birthday parties and weddings—some of life's most cherished moments—out of fear of the food that isn't included in their plan. Complete absurdity.

Egg whites, steamed broccoli, tilapia, and oatmeal every single day gets old. When you eat the same thing daily, it loses its appeal. You can love chicken but eating it 38 times a week may very well ruin chicken for you. You become resentful of food. You crave things but you have been brainwashed to think you can't have something if it's not on the meal plan. A lettuce wrapped avocado and turkey burger is a great meal, but since it's not on your structured meal plan, it's not allowed. This is a problem. You start to think of nutrient dense foods as "bad" just because your meal plan doesn't include them.

Everyone has a breaking point when it comes to a meal plan, whether it's six days, six weeks, or six months. You eventually come to realize that this approach isn't long-term because you see your social life slipping, your energy fading, and you are completely exhausted. You know your diet is too extreme and stressful and you crack. You feel like you have nowhere left to go.

"One of the longer standing debates, with a lot of flip-flopping over the years is whether diets are failing for biological or psychological reasons. Now, first off let me say that the distinction is a false one and you can't ever separate the two: biology affects psychology and psychology affects biology." -Lyle McDonald

Some people never achieve their dream body because they can't stick to a meal for longer than two weeks. Some people last months and months on a plan, make extremely impressive progress, and then lose it because they grow exhausted and can no longer maintain progress. Some people stick to it for years and years because they are extremely disciplined. They have never broken from the plan because they are too afraid to. They envy people who can go out for a celebratory dinner and enjoy dessert with it.

I mentioned previously that you don't need to have a coach holding your hand for the rest of your life. The ultimate goal here is to become an educated and self-governing individual. A structured meal plan keeps you extremely dependent on your coach. You keep going back to your coach, giving that person more money, and all you get in return is a meal plan you know nothing about along with an eating disorder. You are left with no knowledge and you feel lost. No adult should have another adult telling him or her what to eat for an indeterminate amount of time.

By learning how to eat flexibly, you are thinking for yourself. You are learning how to not be controlled by food, because you are in charge. By knowing appropriate food substitutions, and understanding how you can eat doughnuts without any negative consequences, you have the upper hand on food and you are in control, because you are defining the daily parameters of your relationship with it. If you want to eat for life, you need to be willing to learn about nutritional science.

This is not your typical "Get Ripped Quick!" diet book. This book takes into account the oft-neglected psychological aspects of nutrition in order to help you build and maintain a healthier (and more productive) relationship with food. Whether you want to lose weight, keep off the weight you've lost, or perform better, flexible dieting is the best approach.

2. My Story

I think it's important to share my personal relationship history with nutrition and food because it seems like most people can relate in some way.

I grew up with athletic parents in Hawaii. If you have been to the islands, you know the cuisine. Fish, chicken, rice, fresh fruit, etc., and of course fried Spam, though we weren't that Hawaiian. Healthy living and healthy food surrounded me since birth and I understood what foods were good for me and what foods were considered "treats" by my parents. My mother was an excellent role model and I was usually allowed treats in moderation after I finished my well-balanced dinners. When I look back now, I realized that my mom instilled a great relationship with food in me.

It is difficult to pinpoint when my unhealthy relationship with food began, but it was definitely sometime in high school after relocating to Nevada. I started working out at 14 years old and I would hear about nutrition at the corporate gym where my mom was a personal trainer. Many of my parents' friends were involved in competitive bodybuilding and I would often hear them talk about their strict diets, and seeing their phenomenal physiques left my 14-year-old self with the impression that strict meal plans of chicken, fish, greens, brown rice, and oats were the way people had to eat in order to look like that. I recalled the foods I grew up eating with my athletic parents, and it made sense to me, as there were a lot of similarities. Being 14, I didn't understand that getting stage ready for bodybuilding was a very intense and extreme process. It is also the culprit for what a lot of what we call "Bro Science" today.

This was just the beginning of what would be years of severe personal issues with food and nutrition.

I became addicted to cocaine at the age of 16. I would eat maybe once a day, not because of an eating disorder, but because cocaine suppresses appetite. I spent months addicted to cocaine and after my first time getting clean, I gained some unwanted (but much needed) weight. I was dangerously thin and when I cleaned up, the weight gain shocked me. I would do hours of cardio after I ate in hopes of "burning it off". I had replaced a cocaine addiction with a cardio addiction before I graduated high school. This cycle lasted only as long as I could stay clean, which was never long.

The drug use carried over into college. I was always active and fit, but I rarely ate. I spent my first year of college partying and trying to "eat clean" when I did eat. I picked up my first personal training job at the same globo-gym I was a member of for years. If I wasn't exposed to enough garbage nutritional information beforehand, this certainly did the trick. I was a brainwashed drug addict with a dearth of unhealthy behaviors. I took nutrition classes in college so I understood what food did for the human body from a biological and physiological standpoint. I was well-versed in overall nutrition but I knew that college nutrition courses have a purpose of teaching the student about nutritional science and health, not about aesthetics and performance, which were the only two things I cared about until I was 23.

When I cleaned up from my second cocaine addiction in college,

I did what they teach you in rehab: "Stay busy". I chose to stay busy by bodybuilding, which is not the best hobby for an addict, but I thought I had it all figured out since I was a personal trainer. I hired a coach who is now very well known for putting all her clients on cookie-cutter starvation diets. I had to stick to the meal plan, and if I ate an extra ounce of chicken because I was hungry, I would absolutely loathe myself, then punish myself for the transgression. One day my coach (who was prepping for a show herself) told me that she broke down and had cake the night before her show and her coach instructed her to throw it up. This was when things got really bad for me, as I had never previously realized that purging was an "option". I made this my option for years (from roughly the ages of 19-24). I even dated a guy for a year and a half who insisted I regurgitated everything I ate. He liked thin girls and made me feel like I wasn't attractive if I weighed over 130 pounds at 5'8". While I was with him, I was still personal training and I got my FNS certification (Fitness Nutrition Specialist). It was at this point that I actually started learning some decent basic knowledge about nutrition.

After getting my FNS, I was able to better apply what I had learned in a classroom setting in college toward my job and day-to-day life. At this point in time I understood optimal protein intake for active people, discerned that carbohydrates were necessary, firmly believed in clean eating, and I was an advocate of the "cheat meal". My philosophy was better, but far from great. I was still a die-hard "clean eater", but at least I could enjoy a cheat meal without throwing it up afterward (progress, not perfection). I still believed in meal plans, but I wrote lenient ones for all my clients. I gave them lists of food and told them they had meal choices; for example, they could choose fish or chicken along with their choice of greens and pair it with one of the "approved" carbs for lunch and dinner. This was my way of giving my clients the freedom of choice without restricting them, as I knew what it felt like to be on a strict starvation meal plan. They all had a list of approved healthy snacks that they could choose from and they were allowed a cheat meal each week. This is not a bad approach to nutrition per say, especially for someone fairly new to flexible dieting, however there are still too many restrictions. It was essentially a "cookie cutter" plan, albeit less restrictive, as everyone was given the same things, with the only difference being that men received larger portion sizes.

At this point in time I had also decided that gluten and dairy were the roots of all evil and I was one of those self-righteous orthorexics who couldn't associate with anyone who didn't share my nutrition philosophy. This went on for a few years and at the tail end of it, my social media started to take off and I was posting daily pictures of my egg whites with spinach and my scrawny physique (because I was so lean I had a fit appearance, but it was dangerously unhealthy). People were willing to listen to what I had to say.

But the problem was that I was living a lie. I was still using drugs fairly often, I was closet drinking, and I was so nutrient-deprived and malnourished that I would binge after days of minimal calories and repeat the cycle of self-loathing and purging. I would preach "clean eating" and "no excuses" on my social media to an extreme, then resume my unhealthy behaviors in real life.

In 2012, something changed. I discovered functional fitness thanks to Instagram and I was obsessed. With the functional fitness boom of 2012, also came the paleo boom. I switched my diet to a caveman diet: high protein, high fat, and low carb. There were no "rules" other than to eat paleo-approved foods (these aren't the only rules, but that's what everyone thought). Everything revolved around bacon and avocado and there wasn't a grain in sight. I read every paleo book on the market and I convinced myself that I finally knew what I was doing. With the increase in calories from eating paleo, also came an increase in energy. I was eating substantially more than I had in a while and of course, this meant I felt like training more with all the extra energy from healthy foods. I started to strength train daily and sometimes I would train close to 6 hours a day and I looked stronger than I ever had. Was this because I was eating paleo? Absolutely not, but at the time I thought paleo deserved the credit. I looked the way I did because I was eating thousands of calories a day and training excessively because of it, so of course I looked better. I was muscular but I still had a softer look and I was recovering terribly from a lack of carbohydrates. I ate paleo until late 2012 and I occasionally binged on "off limits" foods that I was craving. When I binged, I purged. The unhealthy relationship with food carried on, despite my half assed attempts to "fix" it.

I decided to get a breast augmentation in December of 2012 and I did not prepare for it. When you eat over 3500 calories and train 6 hours a day, you can't just stop doing one of those things and expect to still do the other. The training stopped but the eating and drinking continued. I ballooned up after surgery and I assumed it had to do with swelling from the operation, which amounted to 25 pounds of "swelling" in a month. I looked terrible. That was the first time I ever saw the scale go above 160 pounds… and it reached 182. After I panicked and cried for a day, I slashed my calories and went back to the old "bro diet" of high protein and low fat; I did an hour of cardio a day. I was extreme again. Ten pounds came off in 10 days and I turned to taking illegal substances to get the weight off. These illegal substances are not a good thing to pair with an alcohol problem, and I could feel myself mentally slipping. I found myself angry, insane, and obsessive, along with another handful of bad character traits.

After a few months of this vicious cycle in early 2013, things got worse which led me down a dark path of destruction which brought me to sobriety from everything. No more PEDs, no more alcohol, and no more extremes. I promised myself to live a balanced life. As mentioned before, my "stay sober" method was basically "stay busy" so I chose to do a dietetic internship. I read Lyle McDonald's flexible dieting PDF that was referred to me by another intern in the program, and decided to loosely apply it to myself even though I was extremely skeptical. It went against everything I thought I knew about nutrition. It explained why strict eating does not work and gave the explanation that flexible dieting is a non-strict approach to nutrition. It worked and I was stoked because I was eating doughnuts guilt-free and I was getting stronger while slimming down, but I needed to know more. My interest was piqued, and it was at this time that I found Dr. Layne Norton (who is my nutrition coach and mentor now). I watched all of his videos and soaked up everything I could. I finally realized that if I were to figure out how many calories a day

I needed to consume to support my activity and reach my goals, I could meet my protein requirement and figure out what combination of carbs and fat I needed to get the best results. Enter flexible dieting with macros.

I started out as a strict macro-counter. I got a high from hitting my numbers dead on every single day and I weighed and measured everything that entered my mouth. I was in this 100%. Now let me be extremely candid: this is a sign of an eating disorder. I was obsessing over food and my definition of nutritional success at this time was predicated on hitting my daily macronutrient allowance dead-on. I found myself popping fish oil pills to hit my fat macros (I think I even mentioned that in my previous book). We will go into more detail in a few chapters on who needs to hit their macros dead-on and when. I was again being extreme despite thinking I was "flexible"; strictly counting, tracking, and hitting macros is also a very rigid practice and not exactly "flexible".

I moved to NYC at the end of 2013 and I wanted to get stronger and bigger. I put myself on a pretty hefty "bulk" in 2014 and I went from 165 pounds to 185 pounds by April; not all of this was good weight as I put it on way too quickly. I was training hard and eating big, but I did not feel great at 185 pounds. This is where things really got fun. Since I had "reverse dieted" myself up to eating 2800 calories a day, weight essentially fell off of me when I dropped to 2500-2600 calories a day. I cut to 170-175 very easily with little to no effort and I was thrilled about this. This was the first time I had ever lost weight eating over 2500 calories a day. In September of 2014 I decided to pursue competitive powerlifting.

With my pursuit of powerlifting, I knew that I wanted to drop to a lower weight class and preserve strength (something that is not easy to do without a sound approach to nutrition). I was strong but not strong in comparison to other females at my weight. This was when Dr. Layne Norton started coaching me. I knew that I needed to be held accountable for my nutrition if I was going to cut all the way down to 148, which was the weight class in which I wanted to compete. I had plenty of experience with flexible dieting by this time but minimal experience with cutting to make a weight class. In 14 weeks, I got about 18 pounds off and lowered my BF% to 14%. I did this never eating less than 2300 calories a day. I was extremely consistent and diligent with my nutrition but not to the point of being obsessive. I learned how to be truly flexible and track loosely whilst getting permanent results. I also sacrificed minimal strength and performance since I took the slow approach.

I had finally figured it out. This takes patience and it takes the dieter to realize that perfect is the enemy of good. I was finally seeing the results in myself that my clients had been seeing when working with me, and I give credit to two things: 1) consistency and 2) having someone hold me accountable which was something I had never had. By paying for those 3 months of guidance from Layne, I was able to get the weight off and keep it off. I learned so much about my body and that experience will be with me forever. I have now used flexible dieting to reach every goal imaginable.

In 2014 I was able to work with NFL players, functional fitness athletes, and NPGL athletes. I consider myself a major pioneer of integrating flexible dieting into performance sports. I think it's an excellent way for an athlete to learn what is optimal for their body composition and performance. Being able to determine how many carbohydrates should be consumed daily to maximize athletic potential should be every athlete's goal. Some athletes need to cut weight for a meet or to improve speed and some need to gain weight to improve power. All of these things can be done through flexible dieting.

3. Flexible Dieting & Why Macros Win

Within the context of this book, flexible dieting is an empty vessel, which is to say that it's a term that means what you want it to mean. I know this is extremely ambiguous but I urge you to create your own definition that will best assist you to find success in this. I shared two examples of flexible dieting definitions in the first chapter, and you will see several "interviews" throughout the book where athletes who have adopted flexible dieting share their viewpoints and personal definitions.

Here is another fantastic definition from my friends at Eat to Perform:

"In the most basic sense, flexible eating is a low-stress, open-minded approach to nutrition that includes foods based upon context, not upon labels like "clean," "dirty," "good," or "bad." Whether it be for fat loss, lean mass gain, or to fuel high-intensity exercise, this method looks at the intrinsic value of food choices and emphasizes the big picture rather than assigning foods to a "naughty" or "nice" list irrespective of their effect on your

progress. The positive effects of eating a food are weighed with equal importance to the potential negative effects."

Flexible dieting allows you to set up a diet you can realistically maintain without sacrificing your physique, your relationships, or your sanity. Perfection is not expected; only progress. With this approach, you don't need to justify or vindicate your eating habits. Just eat what you want, when you want to in moderation while remaining in your macro target range.

You undoubtedly see people plaster their social media accounts with cookies, pizza, pancakes, doughnuts, burgers, and all the other foods that we have been conditioned to call "junk". This is extremely flexible dieting and I need you to remember that people are not posting everything they eat. These people are the typical IIFYM-ers who misrepresent flexible dieting for two reasons:

1. They tend to not be educated on the notion that micronutrients (and green things) are necessary for our overall health. They don't understand the importance of food quality or they have poor nutritional knowledge. These are not the people whom you should be seeking nutritional advice from. I don't care how badly you want to eat cereal all day long; you should still eat some fucking vegetables.

2. They know that a plate of chicken and greens is boring so they prefer to get attention for the box of doughnuts or tray loaded with burgers and fries. "Likes", shares, and retweets are more important than sending the right message, oftentimes. Showcasing a ripped six-pack in one social media post then a pizza in the next provides shock value. These people are trying to get a point across but they are forgetting to share the intricate details. There is a lot more to it than "eat doughnuts then do deadlifts" (www.DoughnutsAndDeadlifts.com) #productplacement.

You can absolutely get jacked or lean by eating nothing but non-nutrient dense foods and "hitting" your macros (assuming you have them calculated correctly), but eating this way does not take into account the health of the brain, heart, or other vital organs. Not to mention those participating in performance sports need to be at the top of their game. If you eat processed garbage, you may not see negative repercussions on the outside, but it will be taking a toll on your insides. I prefer the term "flexible dieting" over "if it fits your macros" because that is exactly what it is: an ability to be flexible and non-restrictive with your food choices in order to maintain a healthy lifestyle and achieve your goals.

Your food possibilities are endless; you don't have to eat the same meals day after day if you don't want to, and there is nothing prima facie "off limits". You can indulge in periodic cravings with some simple tracking and planning, and through this process you will begin to develop a healthier relationship with food as opposed to fearing it. Flexible dieting completely goes against conventional dieting, and the notion that anyone who wants to get in shape has to eat a rigorous diet, composed of a narrow number of "clean foods". Flexible dieting countervails the practice to eat at precise times throughout the day, and challenges the fatalist notion that any slight deviation from these oft-cited dietary strictures is akin to "breaking the rules", and thus, tantamount to failure. Flexible dieting is simple: you eat whatever foods you like that fill your allowance of proteins, carbs and fats and the foundation of your diet should be built upon foods that contain a rich micronutrient profile. If you stray from the plan because you are in the mood for a scoop of ice cream, it's OK because you will know how to account for it.

Let's dig a little deeper. In order to be able to mentally handle flexible dieting and macro counting, you need to be able to understand that food is food. Stop looking at fat and carbs as "bad", and instead realize that only certain portions of them are bad. Remember what was discussed in Chapter One, and wipe the concept of "clean eating" from your mind. When you learn the fundamentals of macronutrients and how much of each your body needs, you are in complete control. You learn to be responsible and not overdo it. It seems fitting to quote the Greek philosopher Epicurus who said, "Be moderate in order to taste the joys of life in abundance".

There are no dietary restrictions with counting and tracking macros as long as you are hitting your carefully calculated daily intake. I am going to assume that if you are reading this, you like lead a moderate-to-active lifestyle. Therefore, I can go ahead and assume that you maintain a diet containing plenty of nutrient dense foods. So now it's just a matter of fine tuning and filling up those macros with the right choices and at the right times. You are going to have to put in more work at the start in order to reap the long-term benefits associated with flexible dieting. You will have to read labels, you will have to plan, and you will have to track and count for a little while. The more effort that you demonstrate in the beginning, the easier the long-term approach will become.

Once you are able to recognize that an occasional indulgence will not throw you off track, you suddenly realize that remaining balanced and holding yourself accountable is simple. Once you are able to grasp that 50 grams of carbs is 50g of carbs regardless of the source, you will experience a feeling of freedom unlike any other. Here's an example: a banana is carbs, gummy worms are carbs, bread is carbs, and broccoli is carbs. They are all the same, but don't take that too literally as some are far more rich in micronutrients as discussed earlier. The actual size of what 50 grams of carbs will look like is what will differ, but 50 grams is 50 grams. Both are supplying your body with exactly that. Now naturally the next thing that will pop into your head is sugar, or I as like to call it: "street legal crack cocaine".

We will go into details about carbohydrates, but I will let this marinate in the mean time: if you are meeting your daily fiber goals, it is impossible to consume an excessive amount of sugar. I will say this: If you do get all your calories from "junk", you'll probably feel like junk, definitely not what you want before or after a long training session. Even though 50g carbs is the same whether you consume it by way of processed sugar or by way of green veggies, one is obviously more nutrient dense thus "healthier". What I am trying to teach you, is that occasional leniency with yourself is OK, but too much won't produce a desired outcome for you. Long story short, you don't have to get a week long case of the "fuckits" if you eat some shit. Put those guilt-free calories straight into your training and be pumped about the PR's you're about to hit.

As I previously mentioned, there is a common misconception that macro counting and flexible dieting means eating whatever the hell you want. This couldn't be more false. This isn't a free-for-all bacon wrapped doughnut festival (but if you have a chance to attend one, don't pass it up). Let me put it this way: let's say you are on a 2000-calorie cut and you are consuming 170 grams of protein, 190 grams of carbs, and 65 grams of fat a day. Good luck filling your macros with pastries, french fries, and ice cream. In order to get that much protein, while somewhat restricting carbs and fats, you are going to have no choice but to rely heavily on things like eggs, meat, poultry, potatoes, oats, vegetable, fish, etc., unless you plan on living on protein shakes (have fun with those poops). Sure, you definitely will have some wiggle room for the "fun" stuff each day if you plan ahead and eat right, but don't kid yourself and think that you can spend your days eating endless amounts of everything as a flexible dieter. It doesn't quite work that way; especially when it comes to carbohydrates, as you will see in the next chapter.

Flexible Dieting is Goal Specific and Easily Modified

Being a "flexible dieter" isn't a temporary moniker, or a quick fix diet solution. It's not a 30-day challenge, a 21-day detox, or a 10-day cleanse. Flexible dieting is a lifestyle, one that once permanently adopted can be universally adapted to help you achieve any goal, aesthetic and athletic, that you have now, and in the future.

Fitness and nutrition go hand in hand. Fitness is not a temporary thing, nutrition shouldn't be, either. You have to be active and train year-round, thus you need to have your nutrition in check year-round, as well. You need to go into this with the realization that this may likely amount to a complete lifestyle overhaul. Moreover, these changes need to be lasting. I think you will see that by getting your nutrition on point, you will experience a massive breakthrough with your training. You will be adequately fueled and ready to take on even the most grueling days.

One key thing to remember is the phenomena of adaptation. As you adapt to vigorous training and evolve as an athlete, your diet will need to be adjusted accordingly. As you train more (especially competitively), you may need to eat more. If you lose a lot of weight, there is less mass on your frame and your body will require less food. Conversely, if you gain weight, there is more mass on your frame and your body will likely require more food. You simply add or subtract calories, and with some basic math you can determine the optimal amount of each macronutrient that will best suit you and help you reach your goal efficiently.

When approaching a new goal, you may need to alter your personal set of flexible guidelines to help you better reach that goal. For example, if your goal is to lean out, you may need to tighten up your high-calorie food consumption in order to make sure you don't ever feel hungry. When I am trying to lean out, I limit my "treats" to one a day (unless I have "leftover" macros at the end of the day). When I am at a caloric deficit, I also avoid drinking any calories in the form of protein shakes, smoothies, energy drinks, or sodas. When I am focused on performance, I let myself get away with more calorically dense foods, but try to eat them post-training in order to aid my recovery. I created these guidelines based on past experiences with my clients and myself. When your dietary guidelines change parallel with your goals, you are truly being a flexible dieter.

There is something extremely rewarding about knowing how to properly calibrate your nutrition. Whether it is your own diet or your clients', knowing how to reach an athletic or aesthetic milestone via nutritional knowledge is an invaluable skill that more people ought to have. Educating people that extremes don't need to be taken is a must and those of us in leadership positions need to take charge. By teaching people how to gauge food better, we are setting up long-term success and improving the relationship between the food and the eater.

"Flexible dieters put the magnitude of their mistake into perspective. They realize that one scoop of ice cream or an Oreo has literally delayed their progress by about 100 calories — the equivalent of maybe an hour or two of dieting."–Armi Legge

The wonderful thing about working with athletes, is they understand they need to eat. This is the primary reason as to why I have switched gears. I mentioned on Mark Bell's podcast, "The Powercast", in early 2014 that I was trying to move away from weight loss nutrition and focus primarily on athletes. Unfortunately, many of my past clients took offense to this and thought I was being pretentious. Let me explain:

Losing weight, contrary to popular belief or personal experience, is relatively easy. It's a simple matter of energy balance: eat less, train more, and you will lose weight. The physiological specifics of weight loss are no secret. What is difficult about losing weight are the behavioral and psychological components. Everyone I know has some sort of emotional or mental relationship with food. Many are healthy relationships, but most are not. Being one of those people with a very unhealthy past relationship with food, it was emotionally exhausting for me to talk to fellow disordered people, day in and day out, feeling like I was constantly repeating myself. My best clients got the hang of flexible dieting in two or three weeks, at which point I generally never heard from them again. This meant success to me. People tell me that I am crazy for desiring a high client turnover rate without seeing why from my point of view. Each time a client leaves me because they are able to handle their own nutrition, this means that I have taught them well. Once someone has lost 5 pounds from flexible dieting, they better understand, and trust, the program. The client who actually does everything their coach advises will often lose that 5 pounds in 1-2 weeks (unless of course there are deeply rooted issues from years of metabolic damage).

Aside from previously having an eating disorder, I am not the most qualified person to assist people who are recovering from theirs. Nor am I the most patient when it comes to people who lack consistency and follow-through. Anyone with a healthy mindset who is willing to commit fully to the tenets of flexible dieting will see results simply by reading this book, and applying its principles.

Being an athlete is not easy. You need to be coached if you are going to take your sport seriously. The less you have to worry about nutrition and programming, the more you can focus on the actual training and recovery. I thoroughly enjoy optimizing performance through nutrition. An athlete understands that there is always room for improvement and is willing to do anything to excel. When I prescribe macronutrients to an athlete, he or she doesn't question them or make excuses as to why they aren't following through with them. This makes my job a lot easier because I am not constantly having to chaperone their diets, or remind them when and how to eat.

Another exceptional quality of athletes, is their understanding of timelines. Everyone loves seeing quick results, but there is a certain type of patience that is unique to competitive athletes. They typically eschew short-term solutions; instead, they are looking for a nutritional method that they can utilize for the duration of their careers, not just for a few weeks or months.

I think the real problem is that not enough people consider themselves athletes. I'm a big fan of my good friend (and Critical Athlete co-founder) Matthew Aikin's stance on the matter: "If you played hide-and-go-seek as kid, congratulations! You're an athlete". If you use your body for something more than it's basal functions (breathing, sleeping, sitting), you can rightfully consider yourself an athlete. Perhaps not a competitive one, but an athlete, nonetheless. And athletes don't come in uniform packages. If a person has 100 pounds to lose, this does not mean that he or she isn't athletic, or unsuited to athletic training. Too many people think that all the weight must come off before any serious training can take place, and this is not the case. Strength and performance goals ought to be as important as weight loss goals.

It's unavoidable that different things have to be prioritized at different times (we will go over this in more detail in later chapters), but I think that many people get far too preoccupied with the number on the scale diminishing, and discount the importance of things like improved strength and stamina that are equally laudable measures of success. If your primary goal with flexible dieting is weight loss, and the scale doesn't change one week, it's important to have contingent goals to hold your hat on to forestall premature discouragement. I recommend these contingent goals be capacity, not aesthetically, related.

If you are reading this book because you want to lose weight, I want you to come up with two goals-one primary, the other contingent-before you get underway:

1. How many pounds do want to lose from your frame?

2. How many pounds do you want to add to your back squat, in 12 weeks time?

Even if you don't even lift (bro), feel free to substitute an endurance, or mobility related goal. The point is, make it measurable, and make it matter to your overall health and well-being.

An athlete's body is a byproduct of their training. The efficacy of their training is a byproduct of their nutritional habits. One can't perform adequately without enough of the right foods at the right times. By introducing flexible dieting into performance sports, we can optimize performance by introducing a unique and tailored amount of protein, carbohydrate, and fat to the individual athlete. When you eat to perform, you perform pretty damn well, and it shows from both an athletic and aesthetic standpoint.

We have already discussed how simple it is to calibrate nutrition with flexible dieting in order to produce desired results. Taking an extremely unique approach seems to be ideal with athletes and with a few weeks of trial and error, it proves to be pretty easy to pinpoint precisely how many grams of each macronutrient an athlete should be consuming. Once the precise numbers are determined, the diet basically goes into autopilot and can be easily adjusted if training volume increases or decreases, or if more specific goals come into play.

If you compete in a sport that has a weight class aspect, you can easily and safely cut weight without performance or strength suffering. Dramatic, quick weight loss is the wrong route for making a weight class. The slower the cut, the easier it is for the body to adjust and acclimate to losing mass while still being able to move mass efficiently and powerfully.

Few professional sports possess the demands (or reward as highly) for speed and agility as football (no, I don't mean soccer). Second round draft pick and New York Jets tight end, Jace Amaro, contacted me for nutrition help in 2014. He needed to drop a specific amount of fat in order to improve his performance on the field before the first season of his NFL career got underway. We lowered his body fat by 6% in roughly 8 weeks (that's a considerable amount for someone who is 6'5 and 260 pounds). We did it by determining the optimal protein, carbohydrate, and fat intake for his size, activity, and goals. He also optimized his nutrient timing based off of his two-a-day training of team practices and weight training. My point? This works for everyone. From elite athletes to people who have never worked out a day in their lives.

Lastly, athletes get injured. Every sport has a risk factor to consider and the more active you are, the more likely you are to be injured at some point in time. Flexible dieting can take this into account. In the coming chapters, we will go over your multiplier which is determined by your level of activity. If for whatever reason you become temporarily inactive or less active because of an injury, you can lower your multiplier (and avoid unintended weight gain) until you are ready to get back to training. Unnecessary weight gain is avoidable when you are recovering from injuries or limited in training.

Closing Comments Before the Science and Math

Be flexible with healthy choices; allow treats when your macros permit them. When you expect perfection from yourself, things become too absolute. Being completely absorbed by nutrition causes unneeded stress, which can take away focus and attention that should be going toward the more important areas of your life such as your relationships or your career. By eliminating the stress of what to eat and when to eat it, you free up a lot of cognitive energy that would otherwise be spent obsessing unneededly over your diet, and you feel more at ease.

Complicated nutrition protocols are extremely unnecessary for most people. You do not need to buy a diet book (other than this one, insert winky face emoji).

"Even the books that tell you that you don't have to count calories still ultimately trick you into eating less, by adjusting what you can eat (and sometimes when you can eat it). Low-carbohydrate, low-fat, the Zone, you name a diet and they are making you eat less food in the long run. There's simply no way to escape that, no matter what magic they promise. Other weight loss approaches take the exercise route, get you burning more calories through activity under the assumption that you won't just eat more to compensate (which tends to be a rather bad assumption most of the time). There's really nothing magical to weight loss no matter what you want to believe."
-Lyle McDonald

People are always looking for the perfect regimen of training and nutrition to get the best results, but the problem is that there is no perfect regimen, and you can only determine what is optimal for you. You will exhaust yourself doing a month of research to determine what "diet" you should be on, and that's 30 days you have already wasted. Rather than spending 30 days looking at what other people are doing, I just ask for 30 days of consistency with your macronutrients and training. With 30 days of flexible dieting, you can determine your calorie balance, how big of a surplus or deficit you should be at, and figure out how to get into target range of your daily macronutrient allowances. Say no to nutritional FOMO.

"A good solution applied with vigor now is better than a perfect solution applied ten minutes later." - George S. Patton

That initial 30 days can set you up for an entire year of success. When you look at your diet over the course of a year, it is easier to realize that occasional treats are no threat in the grand scheme of things as long as you are consistent 80-90% of the time. Dietary leniency and flexibility is not a big deal unless you make it one. When you look at your training over the course of a year, it is easier to realize that a lot of detail goes into programming. When you start a new training cycle, you don't expect to put 100 pounds on to your squat in a few weeks, because it takes time to acquire strength and power. If you are able to trust your training program, you can trust the nutrition strategy that supports it. The long term approach is the optimal approach for most people. You can set bigger athletic goals if you look at the quarter, half, or full year as opposed to just weeks or months. Same goes for nutrition. Setting small, incremental goals that aggregate over time into one larger goal is the ideal approach for any athlete. I strongly suggest that you make a 30-day commitment to acclimate to flexible dieting and see the benefits. Afterward, I want you set a year-long goal broken into four, 3-month intermediate goals.

Now lets get into the nitty gritty of how you go about flexible dieting.

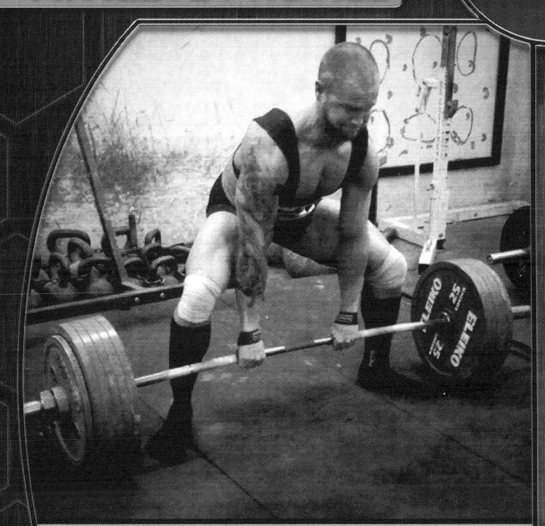

JON STEWART
POWERLIFTING

WHO ARE YOU AND WHAT DO YOU DO?

MY NAME'S JON STEWART AND I'M NOT A TALK SHOW HOST OR RUNNING BACK FOR THE CAROLINA PANTHERS, UNFORTUNATELY. I AM, HOWEVER, A STRENGTH AND CONDITIONING AND NUTRITION COACH BASED OUT OF ALBERTA, CANADA. I SPLIT MY TIME BETWEEN BEING THE STRENGTH AND CONDITIONING COACH FOR THE EDMONTON ESKIMOS OF THE CANADIAN FOOTBALL LEAGUE (CFL) AND AS A COACH AND VICE-PRESIDENT OF THE STRENGTH GUYS; AN ONLINE DISTANCE PERFORMANCE COACHING START-UP. I'M ALSO A COMPETITIVE POWERLIFTER IN THE CANADIAN POWERLIFTING UNION (CPU), AND AN AVID CONSUMER OF BOTH DONUTS AND COFFEE. BASICALLY, I LIFT HEAVY AND TRY TO LOOK GOOD, THEN I HELP OTHERS DO THE SAME.

DEFINE FLEXIBLE DIETING IN YOUR OWN WORDS?

I SEE FLEXIBLE DIETING AS A HOLISTIC APPROACH TO NUTRITION. THE WORD "HOLISTIC" GETS A BAD RAP FROM ITS ABUSE BY THE ALTERNATIVE MEDICINE/FITNESS CROWD THESE DAYS, BUT I'M REFERRING TO ITS ORIGINAL MEANING; "CHARACTERIZED BY THE EFFECT ON THE WHOLE PERSON, TAKING INTO ACCOUNT MENTAL AND SOCIAL AND OTHER FACTORS, RATHER THAN JUST THE PHYSICAL". FLEXIBLE DIETING ALLOWS YOU TO EASILY MODIFY YOUR DIET BASED ON YOUR SPECIFIC GOALS AND PREFERENCES VIA SOME VERY EASY TO FOLLOW PROTOCOLS. THE GENERAL EASE OF THIS APPROACH HAS POSITIVE INFLUENCES AS FAR AS ADHERENCE GOES, WHICH IN THEORY (AND HOPEFULLY IN PRACTICE) WILL ALLOW YOU STICK TO YOUR GOALS FOR THE LONG TERM, REACH THEM FASTER, AND ENJOY THE PROCESS ITSELF. YOU'RE PROBABLY SEEING HOW THIS NOW TIES INTO THE SOCIAL AND MENTAL ASPECTS OF OUR BEING. THE BEST DIET IS THE ONE YOU STICK TO, IF YOU CAN'T STAY ON TRACK…THEN WHAT'S THE USE?

WHEN DID YOU START FLEXIBLE DIETING?

I STARTED FLEXIBLE DIETING AROUND 3 YEARS AGO. IT WAS MORE BY MISTAKE, OR I SUPPOSE EVOLUTION, THAN ANYTHING.

WHAT WAS YOUR DIET LIKE BEFORE FLEXIBLE DIETING?

PRIOR TO FLEXIBLE DIETING I HAD TRIED NEARLY EVERY COMMON "BRO" APPROACH. AS A POWERLIFTER MY GOALS HAD ALWAYS BEEN EITHER ADDING SIZE (HYPERTROPHY) OR PURELY STRENGTH, SO STARTING MY HEADFIRST DIVE INTO POWERLIFTING AT THE AGE OF 15 I OPTED FOR A LESS THAN RIGID PROTOCOL OF 'EAT ALL THE PROTEIN AND LOTS OF CARBS + HEALTHY FATS'. THIS INCLUDED AT LEAST 1.5G PER POUND OF BODYWEIGHT IN PROTEIN, WHICH OF COURSE INCLUDED LARGE AMOUNTS OF RAW EGGS WHITES, TUNA "FRESH" OUT THE CAN, BULK CHICKEN BREASTS, OLIVE OIL, OATMEAL, AND CEREAL. IN FAIRNESS TO ADOLESCENT JON, THIS WAS JUST ABOUT THE ONLY APPROACH AROUND AT THE TIME AND WAS DRAWN MAINLY FROM THE OLD ANIMAL MANUALS AND MUSCLE & FITNESS MAGAZINE.

AFTER MY MOVE FROM THE EAST COAST TO ALBERTA IN 2006 I SPENT A YEAR OR TWO WITH PRECISION NUTRITION FOLLOWING ONE OF THEIR EARLY MEAL PLAN SETUPS, WHICH WAS A DECENTLY ROUNDED "CLEAN" APPROACH. HOWEVER, AS A MEAL PLAN I FOUND IT HARD TO STICK TO AND MANY OF THE FOOD CHOICES SIMPLY WEREN'T FOODS I ENJOYED. AFTER PN I MOVED TO A FLEXIBLE AD LIBITUM DIET AND WORKED TO HIT 1G/POUND OF BODYWEIGHT

IN PROTEIN, 1-2 SERVINGS CARBS, AND A SERVING OF FATS VIA 4-6 MEALS A DAY. IN HINDSIGHT THIS WAS A FAIRLY UNSCRIPTED VERSION OF FLEXIBLE DIETING, BUT WITHOUT THE PRECISE CALCULATION AND REGULATION OF MACROS AND OF COURSE STILL STICKING TO WHAT I BELIEVED TO BE HEALTHY FOOD CHOICES. THIS ALL SET THE STAGE FOR THE FLEXIBLE DIETING APPROACH I WOULD ADOPT LATER ON…

WHAT HAS BEEN YOUR BIGGEST BREAKTHROUGH SINCE FLEXIBLE DIETING?

HARD TO LIMIT THIS TO A SINGULAR EVENT AS CHANGES CAME IN RAPID SUCCESSION. THERE WERE A FEW "AH-HA" MOMENTS THAT LEFT ME WONDERING WHERE MY HEAD WAS BURIED A FEW YEARS PRIOR-BUT THAT'S REALLY PART OF BEING A GOOD COACH; LEARNING FROM MISTAKES, ADMITTING YOU WERE WRONG, AND EVOLVING WITH…OR IDEALLY, AHEAD OF THE TIMES.

ONE OF THE BIGGEST REALIZATIONS WERE CERTAINLY THAT SPECIFIC FOODS WERE NOT THE ENEMY AS WE HAD THOUGHT WITH FATS (SATURATED), MILK PRODUCTS, AND HIGH SUGAR FRUITS (IN BODYBUILDING CIRCLES) THROUGH THE 80-90'S. MOST NOTABLY, THAT WHILE ALL FOODS ARE CERTAINLY NOT CREATED EQUAL, THE DIFFERENCE BETWEEN AN ORGANIC SWEET POTATO AND A SLICE OF BLEACHED WHITE GMO BREAD (OUTSIDE OF MICRONUTRIENT CONTENT) IS REALLY NOT THAT LARGE. I THINK I ATE ORGANIC SPOUTED GRAIN BREAD OUT OF "NECESSITY" MUCH LONGER THAN I'D LIKE TO ADMIT…THOUGH EVENTUALLY IT WAS CLASSIFIED UNDER PREFERENCE RATHER THAN "WHITE BREAD KILLS GAINS".

SECONDARY TO THAT, I THINK REALIZING THAT SHORT TERM PROGRESS NEEDS TO BE REPEATABLE IN ORDER TO CARRY OVER TO LONG TERM GAIN; THIS IS WHERE MOST DIETS FALL SHORT AND WHERE FLEXIBLE DIETING SHINES. BEING ABLE TO EASILY MODIFY YOUR DIET TO FIT BOTH YOUR GOALS AND YOUR LIKES/DISLIKES IS A HUGE PLUS FOR MOST PEOPLE. IF YOU CAN'T REPLICATE YOUR SUCCESSES, OR FIND YOURSELF DOING ALL TOO POPULAR YO-YO, THEN PERHAPS LESS STRICTNESS AND MORE CATERING TO YOUR UNIQUE HABITS AND INTRICACIES IS IN ORDER.

WHAT ARE YOUR THREE MOST IMPORTANT GUIDELINES YOU GIVE YOURSELF?

I'M A POWERLIFTER IN THE MIDDLE OF A WEIGHT CLASS (105KG/231LBS; CURRENTLY 225LBS) SO MY GOALS WORK TOWARDS ME FILLING OUT THAT CLASS VIA A SLOW GAIN IN MASS. GRANTED, I'M NOT IN A RUSH HERE, SO I SIT IN A SMALL SURPLUS FOR ABOUT 80% OF THE YEAR WHICH ALSO ALLOWS ME TO RETAIN RELATIVELY LOW BODY FAT IN THE 9-12% RANGE. GIVEN THESE GOALS, I LIKE TO GIVE MYSELF THE FOLLOWING GUIDELINES:

1. 80%-20% RULE APPROACH TO FOOD SELECTION. I'M NOT IN A DEFICIT AND MY TRAINING IS QUITE DEMANDING AT UPWARDS OF 6, 2-3 HOUR SESSIONS A WEEK. THEREFORE, I PREFER TO LIMIT THE RIGIDITY TO MY TRAINING AND ALLOW MYSELF A FAIR AMOUNT OF LEEWAY WITH REGARDS TO FOOD SELECTION WHICH OFTEN COMES IN THE FORM OF A MODEST AMOUNT OF DONUTS, BURRITOS, AND VIETNAMESE CUISINE. WHEN I RAMP UP TRAINING FOR A CONTEST OR DECIDE ON A MINI-CUT I'LL CLEAN THIS UP TO 90-10 OR EVEN 95-5.
2. BASE AROUND PROTEIN. MY PROTEIN INTAKE SITS AT AROUND 250 GRAMS, AND I TEND TO CONSUME 4-5 MEALS A DAY. IT'S EASIEST FOR ME TO CONSUME THIS AMOUNT VIA EQUAL ALLOTMENTS OF PROTEIN EACH MEAL AND I FIND THIS BEST ACHIEVED BY BASING THE MEAL ITSELF AROUND THAT SOURCE. THAT COULD BE ANYTHING FROM A PROTEIN SHAKE, CHICKEN AND VEGGIES, OR A DOUBLE MEAT BURRITO.

3. MICRONUTRIENTS FIRST. MY LAST MEAL OF THE DAY IS ALSO MY POST-TRAINING MEAL, AND IT TENDS TO FALL INTO THE 5-20% I MENTIONED ABOVE. THE DOWNSIDE OF REFINED FOODS IS OF COURSE THEIR LACK OF MICRONUTRIENT CONTENT AND FIBER, SO I MAKE AN EFFORT TO MAKE MY FIRST 3-4 MEALS RICH IN THESE SO I'M NOT HAVING TO WORRY ABOUT THEM TOO MUCH IN MY LAST MEAL OF THE DAY. THIS ALSO PLAYS A PSYCHOLOGICAL ROLE FOR ME, AS THIS MEAL REWARDS ME AFTER A HARD TRAINING SESSION.

WHAT IS THE BEST PIECE OF ADVICE YOU WISH YOU HAD WHEN STARTING FLEXIBLE DIETING THAT COULD HELP NEWBIES?

IF YOU LIKE IT YOU'LL STICK TO IT, IF YOU DON'T… YOU WON'T. IT'S PAINFULLY SIMPLE. IF WE COME FROM A LACK OF STRUCTURE (TYPICAL AMERICAN SEE-FOOD DIET) AND THROW OURSELVES INTO A "CLEAN" CONTEST PREP DIET WE ARE WITHOUT A DOUBT MORE LIKELY TO EITHER A) FAIL OR B) REBOUND HARD ONCE THAT DIET FINISHES. THE RESTRICTIVE WAY ISN'T ALWAYS THE BEST WAY…WE NEED TO CRUSH THIS LINE OF THINKING.

STOP WORRYING TOO MUCH ABOUT NUTRIENT TIMING OUTSIDE OF THOSE OF YOU WHO ARE ELITE ATHLETES. ACE YOUR PROTEIN TIMING VIA AN EQUAL DISTRIBUTION OF PROTEIN TO EACH OF YOUR 3-5 MEALS, OR WITH A SLIGHT BIAS TOWARDS THE WORKOUT PERIOD. FOCUS THAT ATTENTION ON HITTING YOUR MACROS AND DAILY CALORIES WITHIN 100KCALS, MEET OR EXCEED YOU MICRONUTRIENT GOALS, MEET YOU FIBER, DRINK PLENTY OF WATER…AND MOST IMPORTANTLY TRY SOME NEW RECIPES AND FOODS YOUR ENJOY IN MODERATION WITHOUT ALL THAT HEAVY GUILT.

4. WTF is a "Macro"?

It is important for you understand why you should care about what you put in your body. You surely know that protein is important, but do you know why?

Nutrients are the substances that living organisms require to live, function, and thrive. Nutrients are divided into two categories: macronutrients and micronutrients. Some nutrients are only required in trace amounts thus they are collectively referred to as "micronutrients". Vitamins and minerals fall into this category. Micronutrients play a supporting role in the body's metabolism and help with the continuous, complex chemical reactions in the body that keep it alive.

Unlike micronutrients, macronutrients are required in large quantities. Macronutrients are what the body uses for energy. There are three macronutrients: protein, carbohydrate, and fat. There are entire college semesters and textbooks dedicated to teaching how macronutrients are utilized in the human body, but for the sake of brevity (and scope), I will give a more precise rundown. Before we dive in details about each macro, we must quickly discuss metabolism and calories. I am going to give you a very textbook (and by "textbook", I mean Wikipedia, of course) definition of each. If you're interested in doing further research, please do. You will see clickable links that will direct you to sources that will help you in your extracurricular research.

> "'Metabolism' is the set of life-sustaining chemical transformations within the cells of living organisms. These enzyme-catalyzed reactions allow organisms to grow and reproduce, maintain their structures, and respond to their environments. The word metabolism can also refer to all chemical reactions that occur in living organisms, including digestion and the transport of substances into and between different cells. Metabolism is usually divided into two categories: catabolism, which is the breakdown of organic matter and the harvesting of its energy by way of cellular respiration; and anabolism, which is the process whereby the converted energy produced by catabolism is used to construct components of cells such as proteins and nucleic acids. [...] The speed of metabolism, the metabolic rate, influences how much food an organism will require, and also affects how it is able to obtain that food." [1]

Calories measure the amount of energy each macronutrient will provide our bodies with. Our body metabolizes the calories we consume, a process we informally call the "burn". You've likely said some version of the following: "I need to burn off those calories I ate" or, "I try to burn 600-800 calories in my training each day". The word burn is actually describing the phenomenon of thermogenesis—heat generation occurring in the human body.

There are three types of thermogenesis: diet induced, exercise associated, and non-exercise associated. When you take all three types into account, in

---

[1]   http://en.wikipedia.org/wiki/Metabolism

addition to your BMR (basal metabolic rate), which is the rate at which the body uses energy while at rest to keep its vital functions going (e.g. breathing, blood flow, and body warmth), you establish what is commonly know as your *total daily energy expenditure (TDEE)*. Determining your TDEE will give you an estimate of your total caloric expenditure over a 24-hour period, and provide you a starting point that I call an *estimated caloric baseline*.

Notice I used the word "estimate", not "exact". It's impossible to determine what your exact expenditure is, as it fluctuates daily given a variable level of activity. The goal is to get an accurate measure of your TDEE, create a baseline, then go from there. There are numerous ways to calculate this number and I will share my method in Chapter Five when we talk about *energy balance*.

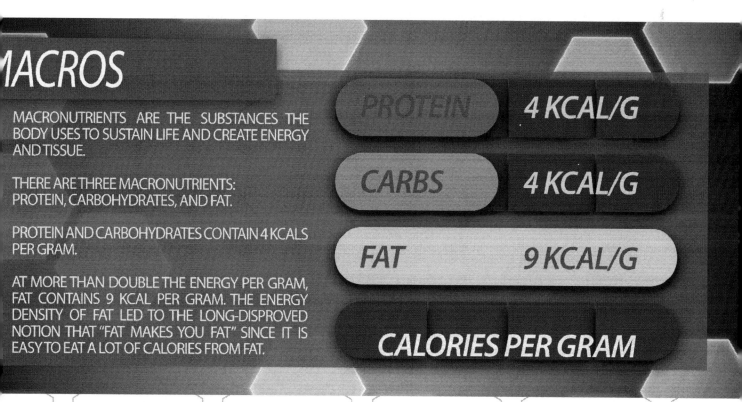

Now that you have a better grasp on calories and metabolism, we can take a closer look at macronutrients and their functions before we start doing math. Yay!

Protein

First and foremost, one gram of protein yields 4 calories. With the basic math you learned in grade school, you can now easily determine how calories x grams of protein is.

Protein is the blanket term for amino acids, which the body requires for a wide variety of functions. Protein is the most essential macronutrient for those who lead an active lifestyle because of the crucial role it plays in muscular growth (hypertrophy) and muscular repair. You've most likely heard protein and amino acids referred to as the "building blocks of the body". When you train, you are breaking down your muscles and you need to consume protein to rebuild them. That being said, protein is considered the superior macronutrient when it comes to body composition.

Protein's function also extends beyond muscle building and repair. Proteins are essential for catalyzing biochemical reactions (enzymes), repairing and replicating your DNA, maintaining immune and cellular function, and cell structure. Biologically, the list goes on; but for our purposes, we want to know its role in shaping how our body looks, works and feels.

It is paramount that you consume enough protein. Inadequate protein consumption will result muscle loss, especially when eating at a deficit. This protein-deficient, muscle-wasting state is called a "catabolic state". This is precisely why protein needs to be prioritized. But just as too little protein can be a bad thing, too much can be detrimental, as well. Excess protein consumption can spike insulin in the same manner as carbohydrates, and chronically elevated insulin levels carry many risks.

It's acceptable to lower fat or carbs when attempting to cut weight or lose fat, but protein is the last macro that should ever be lowered. The only time you should lower protein intake is if you lose a substantial amount of weight.

Lastly, there is a "fee" that the body must pay to digest and absorb food; this is known as the *thermic effect of food (TEF)*. Protein "charges" the most of all three macronutrients, which means that some of the energy we derive from food is lost as heat when it's digested. This in turn promotes weight loss through increased energy expenditure. A protein rich diet can be very helpful during weight loss to maintain lean mass, as well. We will address optimal protein intake in Chapter Nine.

Carbohydrates

Many people call them "The Devil"; I call them "Human Gasoline", with each gram yielding 4 calories.

I'm about to tell you something that may startle you. Are you sitting down?...

Life requires energy.

When we engage in activities that require energy (like living), carbs provide that energy. I said protein is the most important, but carbs are typically the macro that athletic people need the most. If you are training hard, you need ample carbs in order to perform optimally, as they are the most readily used by the body. Anaerobic metabolism prefers to run on glucose, not on fat. If you have no glycogen to utilize during training, your body will automatically recruit amino acids as a back up. Combine this with intense, demanding training and the result will be muscle loss. Not to mention your workouts will blow. Low-carb diets usually mean that you have minimal glycogen needed to maintain strength, speed, agility, and other qualities necessary for optimal performance.

Moreover, long-term carb restriction damages a healthy, functioning metabolism, and is often the culprit for post-diet weight gain.

Every tissue and cell in the body use glucose for energy. Our central nervous system, our heart, our brain, our muscles, and our organs are all dependent upon carbohydrates in order to function properly. We need them for intestinal health and proper waste elimination. Not only do we need carbs to perform physically, but also to perform mentally. Our brains need fuel, too, and it's a very greedy bastard when it comes to glucose consumption. With that in mind, let's talk about cognitive function. Sure, lowering carbs to dangerously low numbers will result in quick weight loss, but it carries unintended consequences. Research has shown that low-carb diets dramatically impair cognitive function. A study from Tufts University shows that when dieters eliminate carbohydrates from their diets, they perform poorly on memory-based tasks compared to dieters on a reduced-calorie diet with adequate carbohydrate consumption. When carbohydrates were reintroduced, cognitive skills normalized.

"While the brain uses glucose as its primary fuel, it has no way of storing it. Rather, the body breaks down carbohydrates into glucose, which is carried to the brain through the bloodstream and used immediately by nerve cells for energy. Reduced carb intake should thus reduce the brain's source of energy. Therefore, researchers hypothesized that diets low in carbohydrates would affect cognitive skills."[2]

Whether you are an athlete, a parent, or a student, you need to be cognitively functional for obvious reasons.

Carbs are also in charge of secreting insulin—an anabolic hormone that has profound effects on tissue growth. Now when I say tissue I mean muscle and fat. When we consume carbs, we use what is immediately needed as insulin binds to receptors on the surface of the muscle. Leftover carbs get stored in our liver and muscle as glycogen to be used later when energy is needed. It's when we consume beyond what is needed that unwanted weight

---

2   Tufts University. (2008, December 15). Low-carb Diets Can Affect Dieters' Cognition Skills. ScienceDaily. Retrieved February 6, 2015 from www.sciencedaily.com/releases/2008/12/081211112014.htm

gain occurs. The goal is to find the "sweet spot" based on our individual needs. There is no magic number when it comes to carb prescriptions, and it's not a "one size fits all" approach.

When we lower carbohydrates, we are lowering more than just calories. Water and carbs have a co-dependent relationship: carbohydrates bind to water, so a decrease in the former create a decrease in the latter. This drop in excess water weight, or "bloat", as the ladies like to call it, is responsible for most of the initial weight loss that occurs after a massive slash in carbs.

Even if carbs are cut extremely low, it's technically possible to produce glucose through gluconeogenesis. The issue here is that you are forcing your body to make glucose from protein opposed to carbs. When this occurs, a bulk of your daily protein consumption is reallocated to energy production rather than muscle growth and repair. If you work out regularly, this poses a problem.

What am I getting at? Eat carbs, please.

Carbs unfortunately, and undeservedly, have a very bad reputation. If you stay under your maintenance calories and are consuming the proper amount of protein, no amount of carb consumption that stays within your caloric range will make you gain weight. If you weight train and stay close to the correct amount of carbs you should be consuming each day, you can reasonably get away with eating the "fun carbs", aka sugar.

Carbs are broken down into simple and complex forms. Simple carbs are fast digesting and easily broken down for immediate energy use. Simple carbs are more commonly known as sugar. Complex carbs are substantially more difficult for our bodies to digest. They are broken down gradually and released into the bloodstream at a slower place. We also have fiber to consider, a certain type of carbohydrate our bodies can't digest (which is a good thing, because it's the engine that drives the poop train).

Foods that are rich in fiber are typically not calorically dense. These foods will allow you to eat a large volume of food without consuming a lot of calories (think leafy greens and other veggies). Because fibrous foods are complex carbohydrates, they are slower digesting and will help you remain full, longer. Fiber also has health benefits for diabetics because it helps to regulate blood sugar. It can also lower cholesterol and help prevent certain types of cancers.

On the other hand, **do not** attempt to fill your entire carb intake for the day by eating a shit load of fiber (pun intended) in the form of green vegetables. They are extremely difficult for your body to break down and believe it or not, you will begin to feel sluggish because too much energy is going into breaking down your food. You will notice digestive discomfort and dysfunction if you are consuming an excess of fibrous vegetables. Excessive fiber intake can oftentimes be worse than inadequate intake (there are countless articles you can find on this with a quick googles search). Aim for 25-40 grams depending on your size and carb intake. Take note that fiber *is* included in your total daily carbs allowance. You are not counting "net carbs"; you are counting your actual total carbohydrate intake, which is made up of fiber, sugar, and starch. Therefore, do not subtract your fiber from your total carbohydrate intake.

There is an entire chapter dedicated to food choices where we will go over how to go about picking the right carb sources for yourself based on hunger levels, daily caloric intake, convenience, cravings, and training time.

Long story short: carbs are the easiest macro to adjust when it comes to flexible dieting. You eat more when you want to gain strength or size, and you eat less when you need to drop weight. We will go over how to precisely and intelligently do this in Chapter Nine as you can't exactly "wing it" until you have spent some time with flexible dieting. We will also discuss "carb cycling" and the role it plays in an active lifestyle.

Fat

One gram of fat yields 9 calories. This is the most calorically dense macronutrient, which is a fact, not a value statement. Do not be afraid of fat. Fat is delicious and easy to include in your diet. No one has ever complained about having to sauté something in butter. Maybe vegans. Ignore them.

Fat, along with carbs, have been regular scapegoats of nutritional fearmongering. Fat does not make you fat. Fats are essential and crucial for our bodies to function at optimal levels. We need fat to survive. We need fat for growth and development, for a secondary source of energy, to maintain cell membranes, and to absorb fat-soluble vitamins. Healthy skin and hair are products of a diet rich in fat. Fat provides cushioning for our organs and joints (and occasionally, the pushin'). Essential fatty acids can't be synthesized by the human body, which means they must be ingested by way of food. Last, but definitely not least, fat is necessary for hormonal balance.

Fat is extremely satiating which means it's great for weight loss. When you are at a caloric deficit, fat is a great way to keep the accompanying hunger pangs at bay, since it is slow-digesting and gratifying to the palate. Fat sits in your stomach much longer than carbs, which is why it is well known for dampening hunger.

As is the case with protein and carbs, some choices of fat are better than others. Some fats (saturated, poly and monounsaturated) are beneficial to our health, while others (trans fats or "hydrogenated" fats) are potentially harmful. Making intelligent food and fat choices will be covered in detail later on.

Now that you have some basic knowledge of the functions of protein, carbohydrate, and fat, it is important to understand that you can calculate, tweak, and calibrate each macronutrient to achieve virtually any aesthetic or athletic goal.

Sources & Further Reading Suggestions:

Westerterp KR, author. Diet Induced Thermogenesis. Nutr Metab (Lond) [Internet]. 2004 Aug 18;1(1):5 Available from: http://www.ncbi.nlm.nih.gov/pubmed/15507147

Michael W King, PhD, author. Gluconeogenesis: Endogenous Glucose Synthesis [Internet] themedicalbiochemistrypage.org. Last modified: January 27, 2015 Available from: http://themedicalbiochemistrypage.org/gluconeogenesis.php

Phillips SM1, Moore DR, Tang JE, authors. A Critical Examination of Dietary Protein Requirements, Benefits, and Excesses in Athletes [Internet]. Int J Sport Nutr Exerc Metab. 2007 Aug 17 Suppl:S58-76. Available from: http://www.ncbi.nlm.nih.gov/pubmed/18577776

Ferris Jaber, author. Does Thinking Really Hard Burn More Calories? [Internet] Scientific American. 2012 July 18. Available from http://www.scientificamerican.com/article/thinking-hard-calories/

Peter Attia, M.D., author. Ketosis – advantaged or misunderstood state? (Part I) [Internet] The Eating Academy, Accessed 2015 January 31 Available from: http://eatingacademy.com/nutrition/ketosis-advantaged-or-misunderstood-state-part-i

Tufts University. (2008, December 15). Low-carb Diets Can Affect Dieters' Cognition Skills. ScienceDaily. Retrieved February 1, 2015 from www.sciencedaily.com/releases/2008/12/081211112014.htm

Chaput JP, Drapeau V, Poirier P, Teasdale N, Tremblay A , authors. Glycemic Instability and Spontaneous Energy Intake: Association With Knowledge-Based Work [Internet]. Psychosom Med. 2008 Sep 7 0(7):797-804 Available from: http://www.ncbi.nlm.nih.gov/pubmed/18725427

Brinkworth GD, Buckley JD, Noakes M, Clifton PM, Wilson CJ. Long-term Effects of a Very Low-Carbohydrate Diet and a Low-Fat Diet on Mood and Cognitive Function. Arch Intern Med. 2009;169(20):1873-1880. doi:10.1001/archinternmed.2009.329 http://archinte.jamanetwork.com/article.aspx?articleid=1108558

Langfort J, Zarzeczny R, Pilis W, Nazar K, Kaciuba-Uscitko H., authors. The effect of a low-carbohydrate diet on performance, hormonal and metabolic responses to a 30-s bout of supramaximal exercise [Internet]. Eur J Appl Physiol Occup Physiol. 1997 76(2):128-33. Available from: http://www.ncbi.nlm.nih.gov/pubmed/9272770

ATHLETE PROFILE

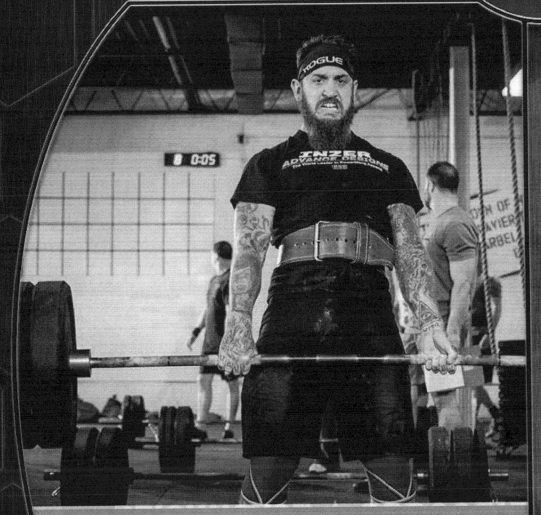

CODY ABELL
CROSSFIT/STRONGMAN

CODY ABELL

WHO ARE YOU AND WHAT DO YOU DO?

MY NAME IS CODY ABELL AND I AM TATTOOER IN VIRGINIA.
I COMPETE IN CROSSFIT AND STRONGMAN.

WHEN DID YOU START FLEXIBLE DIETING?

I DECIDED TO GIVE IT A SHOT AROUND 6 MONTHS AGO.

WHAT WAS YOUR DIET LIKE BEFORE FLEXIBLE DIETING?

I HAD A VERY TYPICAL "CLEAN" DIET OF CLASSIFYING FOODS AS "GOOD" OR "BAD". ONCE A WEEK I WOULD HAVE ALL OUT GORGE AND EAT ICE CREAM, PIZZA, SODA AND WATCH BREAKING BAD. I'D WAKE UP AND FEEL LIKE A PILE OF GARBAGE. IT WAS UNHEALTHY BEHAVIOR AND CAUSING ME TO BE UNHAPPY.

WHAT HAS BEEN YOUR BIGGEST BREAKTHROUGH SINCE FLEXIBLE DIETING?

REALIZING THAT IF I WANT A SNICKERS, ALL I HAVE TO DO IS BE ACCOUNTABLE BY TRACKING IT. FLEXIBLE DIETING HAS RELIEVED ME OF ALL DIET RELATED STRESS, WHICH HAS ALLOWED ME TO FOCUS ON MY TRAINING AND RECOVERY. FLEXIBLE DIETING HAS ALSO ALLOWED ME TO MAINTAIN DIETARY DISCIPLINE LONGER THAN I EVER HAVE IN MY ENTIRE LIFE. IT HAS ALLOWED ME TO HAVE AN ATHLETIC CAREER.

WHAT ARE YOUR THREE MOST IMPORTANT GUIDELINES YOU GIVE YOURSELF?

1. BE PASSIONATE.
2. BE CONSISTENT.
3. BE PATIENT.

WHAT IS THE BEST PIECE OF ADVICE YOU WISH YOU HAD WHEN STARTING FLEXIBLE DIETING THAT COULD HELP NEWBIES?

YOU STILL WANT A SOLID FOUNDATION OF WHOLE FOODS AS YOUR DIET. BUT HAVING A SNICKERS BAR OR A SLICE OF PIZZA OR A SCOOP ICE CREAM WILL NOT DESTROY YOUR DIET AND MIGHT HELP YOU KEEP YOUR SANITY AND ALLOW YOU TO STAY ON TRACK FOR MUCH LONGER

ADDITIONAL COMMENTS:

LIFE ISN'T HARD. LIFE ISN'T EASY. LIFE IS LIFE. YOU ARE RESPONSIBLE FOR THE QUALITY OF YOUR LIFE. SHAPE IT. MOLD IT. TAKE OWNERSHIP OF IT.

5. *Calorie Balance & Finding A Caloric Baseline*

Calorie balance, in short, is the balance of calories consumed versus calories expended. If you are eating more than you are burning, you will gain tissue; if you are burning more than you eat, you will lose *tissue*. Take note of the word tissue. I used that word specifically because weight loss (or gain) is never exclusively fat or muscle, it is always a combination of the two. As mentioned in previous chapters, when it comes to weight loss, the goal is to optimize your diet in order to minimize the loss of muscle tissue and maximize the loss of fat tissue. Now, flip-flop that order (*minimizing* fat tissue while *maximizing* muscle tissue) if you want to board the Gain Train Express, #choochoo. However, you can't optimize anything until you get a grasp of your caloric baseline.

People have argued over optimal nutrition strategies for years, but there is widespread consensus that consistently consuming a *specific* amount of calories (which will vary from person to person) must take precedent. All macronutrient ratio and percentage debates aside, determining your daily caloric intake is the first, and *most important* step, in order to see the benefits for both your physique and performance. There is no sense in obsessing over the *perfect* macronutrient breakdown until you have a general idea of how many calories you should be taking in on a daily basis. Moreover, there is no such thing as a perfect macronutrient breakdown. Don't bother chasing that horizon.

Nick Shaw and Dr. Mike Israetel of Renaissance Periodization give an excellent explanation of why calorie balance is crucial above all else:

> *"Calorie balance is THE MOST important variable in body composition diet success for a very simple reason: it has the greatest impact on how much muscle you can gain and how much fat you can lose over any period of time. It has this powerful impact because of the straightforward fact that calories via fats, proteins, and carbs, literally COMPOSE body tissues. That is, before any muscle can be built, the raw materials (calories from protein, for example) quite literally need to be there, as nothing more than building blocks. On the other end, burning fat requires that not enough calories are shuttled into fat cells to keep them the same size as they lose their fat stores when sending them out into the blood."*[3]

As mentioned in the previous chapter, the first step is to determine your TDEE (total daily energy expenditure) to establish you estimated caloric baseline. Your TDEE will give you a good estimate of how many calories a day you must consume to achieve a neutral caloric balance, which will maintain your current weight and fuel your current lifestyle. Many lifestyle factors, from your training frequency to your day job, need to be taken into account. Two different people who are the same body weight can be on the exact same training program, but if one sits at a desk all day and one cleans houses, the former is going to have a lower expenditure than the latter. Someone who chases kids around all day usually expends more energy than someone who

3   http://www.store.jtsstrength.com/resources//the-renaissance-diet

doesn't. Enter stage left, the lifestyle multiplier.

The multiplier is a far simpler way to calculate your caloric baseline compared to other, more complex metabolic equations. You simply take your current weight in pounds and multiply it by your lifestyle multiplier.

Determining Your Lifestyle Multiplier

This is the part that most everyone overcomplicates. There is absolutely no need to have an anxiety attack over this part. I am going to lay it out for you as simply as possible. Your lifestyle multiplier is going to take into account your training, your job, and your overall level of activity. When you look at these numbers, be honest and realistic with yourself. Rather than choosing the best-case scenario, choose a number that will allow consistency. Accuracy in your choice will yield the best results. Before selecting your multiplier, you need to know that this number is not set in stone... it will change as your training does, it may change if you get a new job, it may change if you get injured, so on.

> **11:** Appropriate for individuals who are virtually sedentary. You may be sedentary for a variety of reasons: a lack of interest or desire to work out, or maybe you're recovering from surgery or a prolonged illness, or a sports-related injury. If you don't partake in strenuous activity at all during the week, you will fall into this category. A lot of grad students tend to get stuck in this category (don't worry, smarty pants. An advanced degree is worth the time).

> **12:** Appropriate for individuals who train less than 5 hours a week. If you make it to the gym a few times a week and train no longer than an hour, you will most likely fall into this category. This multiplier is ideal is for the moderately active person.

13: Appropriate for individuals who train 5-10 hours a week. Most people will fall into this (or the previous) category. You go to the gym during the week for a little over an hour a day and remain relatively active on the weekends.

14: Appropriate for individuals who train 10-15 hours a week, either as longer sessions done 5-6 days a week. Those really dedicated to fitness (but not necessarily training for a specific sport) usually fall into this category. A lot of bodybuilders fall into this category.

15: Appropriate for individuals who train 15-20 hours a week, typically in-season competitive athletes, or people prepping for a meet or competition whose increased training volume warrants a higher multiplier. A lot of people who train twice a day also fall into this category. Many competitive functional fitness athletes, powerlifters, Olympic weightlifters, and strongmen will find themselves here.

16: Appropriate for individuals who train over 20 hours a week for their particular sport. These are typically going to be elite endurance, performance, and strength athletes, oftentimes performing multiple training sessions over the course of a day. Think ultrarunners, competitive cyclists, professional athletes, and Olympians.

***If you are a coach or personal trainer, try to take into account how active you are with your clients. If you tend to train with them or partake in any classes you teach, you may need a higher multiplier because your job could be considered training.

***If you have an active job, but don't think it's enough to justify a higher multiplier, it's OK to add a 0.5 to any of the above numbers. For instance, if your job requires you to be on your feet all day, it may not be enough to bring you up a whole multiplier, but it's probably enough to bring you up a half.

Now this is where I get people asking questions like: "*What if I walk my dog for 30 minutes everyday?*"…"*What if I just do yoga?*"… "*What if I get sick?*"… "*What if I have my kids every other week and I am only active when I have them?*"… What if, what if, what if. Try not to obsess. To reiterate, the goal here is to be flexible, and in doing so build a healthier relationship with food. Take into account everything you have learned up to this point and make an educated choice when it comes to the multiplier that will best suit you. If you do the math for a few different numbers, you will notice that there isn't too big of a difference in the range of estimates.

Once you've settled on a lifestyle multiplier, multiply that number by your body weight to find your caloric baseline, which is the total number of calories you need to consume on a daily basis to maintain your current weight. If you are easily seduced by the prospect of instant gratification, I **strongly** caution against the "slash and burn", cut-all-the-calories-overnight approach. That's counterproductive (and self-destructive) thinking. You are gradually shifting the way you interact with food to bring about positive, and lasting, changes. Drastically cutting calories is a no-no. Remember, the slower the progress, the more permanent the reward.

Now that you have roughly calculated your caloric baseline, you have two options to choose from:

1. Verify your baseline by eating at maintenance for a couple of weeks.

2. Dive straight into eating a deficit (or surplus).

If this is your first foray into flexible dieting, I suggest Option 1. Try it out for two weeks, and if your weight remains stable, you've likely found an accurate caloric baseline. It's important that you don't skip this step in your zeal to start losing weight. It is less costly to take two weeks and verify your caloric baseline, than it is to find out a month later that you've been eating at too small (or large) a deficit, at which point you'll have to start back at step one. There is one minor drawback to this approach, which is that you will need to step on the scale a few times a week to monitor any changes in your weight. If you have a bad history with scales, please be careful with this step. The scale is not a measure of your progress, your potential, or your self worth, it is simply verifying a number for you.

If you find in those first two weeks that you dropped weight, your caloric baseline is slightly higher than you anticipated. If instead you gained weight, you may need to lower your lifestyle multiplier to reflect a lower-than-anticipated caloric balance. If drastic weight change happens in either direction, it may be in your best interest to contact a coach who can assess you and help you get on track. Once you complete Opinion 1, you can move on to Option 2.

If you calculate your caloric baseline, have been flexible dieting for some time, and you have a good idea as to what you maintain on, go ahead and skip to Option 2 by deciding which caloric state will achieve your goal.

Three Caloric States

Maintenance. Also called a eucaloric state, is ideal for anyone who wants to improve body composition while maintaining their current weight. With extreme nutritional precision and specifically programmed training, it is possible to increase muscle tissue and decrease fat tissue over a period of time. Although it is a very slow, difficult, and complicated process, it is possible. This is a great option for competitive athletes who are sitting at a comfortable weight, and have the time to allow their body to adapt slowly to a new maintenance diet.

Deficit. Also called a *hypocaloric* diet, this is going to result in tissue/weight loss. This is more commonly known as a "cut". Since you are taking in fewer calories than you expend, you are forcing your body to burn off extra weight via the utilization of fat (and to a lesser extent, muscle) stores for energy. If weight loss is your primary goal, you should be eating at a caloric deficit. There are many reasons why one may want or need to lose weight, but the *why* is not pertinent when it comes to your calories. All that should initially matter is that you are eating below maintenance.

Surplus. Also called a *hypercaloric* diet, this is going to result in tissue/ weight gain. This is more commonly known as a "bulk". A positive calorie balance means you are ingesting above what you need to maintain, thus the calories are stored as muscle (if you are training) or fat (if you are sedentary). Eating at a surplus is ideal for those wanting to put on mass or beginners who want to make extreme strength or performance gains, which we will discuss in detail.

The following chapters encompass the three caloric states and go into further detail on how to properly and strategically approach each.

Before You Select Your State

There are a few things you need to keep in mind before you decide which of the the three aforementioned states will work best for you. First of all, it is imperative that you avoid enormous shifts in caloric intake. Subtle caloric manipulations are much easier on your body and won't wreak havoc on your metabolism. Be gradual with your approach; different goals will require different phases of calorie balance, but you should never go immediately from a 600 calorie cut to a 600 calorie bulk, or vice-versa. These extremes will consequently lead to a roller-coaster of weight (and emotional) fluctuation. Adding, or subtracting, large amounts of calories to your diet at once is unnecessary and detrimental to your overall well being. Regardless of the route you followed in the past (remembering that as your goals change over time, your nutrition will need to change with them), you should be within the margins of what is a sustainable approach for *you*. If you put yourself on a cut that is setting you up for meltdown to rival Chernobyl, you are not dieting safely within the confines of your chosen caloric state (or reason, for that matter).

The gluttonous, id-driven aspects of our personalities sometimes pressure us to give in to the hedonistic, dietary free-for-all known as a "*dirty bulk*", especially if we've been frustrated by past efforts to gain significant amounts of mass. But a massive surplus of calories doesn't always yield massive gains for everyone. Unless you don't mind gaining some noticeable fluff, a bulk should be carefully planned and regulated. On the other end of the extreme-continuum, we have the *starvation diet*, which I also strongly advise against. If you dramatically cut calories right away, you are left with virtually nowhere to go when an inevitable plateau hits since you are already operating at a sizable deficit. The slower you lower calories, the more gradual the weight loss you are likely to experience, which is preferable because you are left with a lot more wiggle room in which to make adjustments. Lastly, when choosing a caloric state, understand that **you are not stuck** in this state and you can choose to be in a different one at any point in time by simply adding or subtracting calories accordingly. The canvas of flexible dieting remains the same, but you can paint it any color you want. As previously discussed, flexible dieting can be easily adjusted based on current and evolving goals. Over time, as you move through different phases, a foundation of sound principles and practical application will make any modifications or tweaks you make to your diet much simpler, less disruptive, and more effective.

Now let's take a closer look at all three states and determine how to optimize each on an individual basis.

Sources & Further Reading Material

Kevin D. Hall, Steven B. Heymsfield, Joseph W. Kemnitz, Samuel Klein, Dale A. Schoeller, and John R. Speakman, authors. Energy balance and its components: implications for body weight regulation [Internet] American Society of Nutriionists. Am J Clin Nutr April 2012 vol. 95 no. 4 989-994. Accessed at:

http://ajcn.nutrition.org/content/95/4/989.full

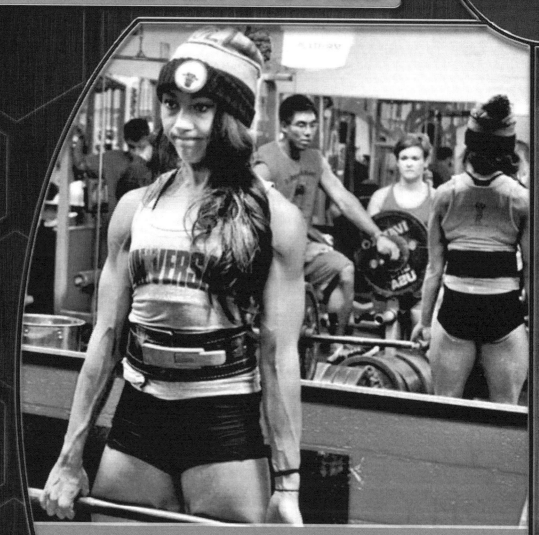

LEANNA CARR
POWERLIFTING/FIGURE COMPETING

LEANNA CARR

WHO ARE YOU AND WHAT DO YOU DO?

MY NAME IS LEANNA CARR AND I'M 23 YEARS OLD. I'M A WNBF PRO FIGURE COMPETITOR AND A RAW 63KG POWERLIFTER IN THE USAPL/IPF.

WHEN DID YOU START FLEXIBLE DIETING?

THREE AND A HALF YEARS AGO, WHICH IS ALSO WHEN I STARTED POWERLIFTING. I'VE BEEN A FLEXIBLE DIETER FROM THE BEGINNING!

WHAT WAS YOUR DIET LIKE BEFORE FLEXIBLE DIETING?

IT RESEMBLED THE TYPICAL COLLEGE STUDENT WHICH INEVITABLY LED ME TO GAIN THE FRESHMAN FIFTEEN (OR IN MY CASE 25). IT WOULD FLUCTUATE BETWEEN PERIODS OF ENTIRELY TOO MUCH TACO BELL AND CHEAP TEQUILA WITH PERIODS OF CRASH DIETING/RESTRICTION/JUICE CLEANSES. TO SUM IT UP, IT WASN'T HEALTHY!

WHAT HAS BEEN YOUR BIGGEST BREAKTHROUGH SINCE FLEXIBLE DIETING?

WELL SINCE I INITIALLY STARTED MY "FITNESS JOURNEY" UNDER THE GUIDANCE OF KNOWLEDGEABLE COACHES (MATT JANSEN AND BRIAN MINOR OF INOV8 ELITE PERFORMANCE) I CAN SAY THAT FLEXIBLE DIETING HAS PLAYED A SIGNIFICANT ROLE IN EVERY ACCOMPLISHMENT I'VE ACHIEVED THUS FAR. NOT ONLY HAS MY BODY COMPOSITION CHANGED COMPLETELY, BUT I'VE BEEN ABLE TO ENDURE STAGES OF MUSCLE GROWTH AND COMPETITION PREP THROUGH FLEXIBLE DIETING, WHICH ULTIMATELY LED ME TO WIN MY NATURAL FIGURE PRO CARD THIS PAST SEASON. IT'S ALSO HELPED ME CONTINUOUSLY INCREASE STRENGTH IN ALL "BIG THREE" LIFTS. I CURRENTLY HOLD THE GA STATE RECORDS FOR MY WEIGHT/AGE IN THE USAPL, I'VE WON NUMEROUS COMPETITIONS, AND ALSO PLACED TOP 5 THIS PAST SUMMER AT MY FIRST RAW NATIONALS POWERLIFTING MEET!

WHAT ARE YOUR THREE MOST IMPORTANT GUIDELINES YOU GIVE YOURSELF?

1. EAT FOR PERFORMANCE. MY MEALS ARE STRUCTURED AROUND MY TRAINING AND I MAKE SURE TO EAT PLENTY OF WHOLE FOODS TO MEET MY MICRONUTRIENT GOALS AND DAILY FIBER REQUIREMENTS.

2. MEAL TIMING. I TIME MY MEALS AROUND MY WORKOUTS. I MAKE SURE TO GET PLENTY OF FOOD, CARBS SPECIFICALLY, BEFORE AND AFTER MY WORKOUTS FOR OPTIMAL FUEL AND RECOVERY.

3. ENJOYMENT. I HAVE A HUGE SWEET TOOTH THAT'S HARD TO NEGLECT! THANKS TO FLEXIBLE DIETING, I DON'T HAVE TO! AT THE END OF THE DAY, MY DIET NEVER FEELS LIKE A DIET BECAUSE IT'S NOT RESTRICTIVE AND I'M ABLE TO ENJOY THE ABILITY OF FLEXIBILITY AND MODERATION!

LEANNA CARR

WHAT IS THE BEST PIECE OF ADVICE YOU WISH YOU HAD WHEN STARTING FLEXIBLE DIETING THAT COULD HELP NEWBIES?

BE PATIENT, ENJOY THE PROCESS, AND DON'T EXPECT TO BE PERFECT. RESULTS WON'T HAPPEN OVERNIGHT AND IT CERTAINLY WON'T BE A PROGRESSIVELY LINEAR JOURNEY. HOWEVER, AS LONG AS YOU'RE CONSISTENT AND ENJOYING WHAT YOU DO, YOU'LL REACH YOUR GOALS AND BE ABLE TO SUSTAIN THEM!

WHAT IS YOUR PERSONAL DEFINITION OF FLEXIBLE DIETING?

EATING FOR A GOAL AND SUSTAINABILITY. AS A PHYSIQUE ATHLETE AS WELL AS A STRENGTH ATHLETE, FOOD IS AN ESSENTIAL PART OF WHAT I DO. NOT ONLY THAT, BUT AS A HUMAN BEING, FOOD IS AN ESSENTIAL PART OF LIFE (DUH). IT IS MEANT TO BE ENJOYED, FUEL OUR BODIES FOR EVERY DAY TASKS, AND IN MY CASE, GIVE ME THE POWER TO SQUAT 2.5 TIMES MY BODY WEIGHT ON THE REGULAR. FLEXIBLE DIETING HAS GIVEN ME THE KNOWLEDGE AND ABILITY TO UNDERSTAND THE CALORIC DEMANDS OF MY BODY, FILL MY BODY WITH PLENTY OF MICRONUTRIENTS FOR OPTIMAL PERFORMANCE, AND MOST IMPORTANTLY, IT GIVES ME THE OPTION OF VARIETY SO I CAN ENJOY THIS LIFESTYLE AND THE OCCASIONAL DOUGHNUT... GUILT-FREE (AS LONG AS IT FITS MY MACROS!)

6. Eating At Caloric Balance (Maintenance)

As you already know, eating at maintenance means you are matching your calories consumed with your calories burned. Because you are in a balanced state, your mass will remain constant. However, if your weight is staying the same, this is not necessarily an indicator that your body composition isn't changing; especially if you are on a very demanding, high volume training program. The tissues being used will correspond to the tissues being built, hence minimal (if any) weight fluctuation.

When eating at maintenance it is important to remember there may be days where you expend slightly more than you took in because you skipped breakfast, or life got in the way and you had to skip a training session. That being said, precise caloric balance is the equivalent of searching for a unicorn. Don't expect it to find it. It's helpful to look at eating at maintenance from an aggregate view, where minor hiccups are ultimately balanced against several weeks of consistent eating. Being too absolute isn't a good thing when it comes to nutrition. Balance is key if the goal is to create a healthy balance, psychologically and physically.

Eating at maintenance is ideal for most seasoned and elite athletes. Demanding exercise is dependent upon steady caloric intake in order for the body to remain in a state of homeostasis:

> *"The concept of homeostasis is an absolutely vital one. To understand it is to understand how organisms can live in a wider range of environmental settings. It also provides the understanding for how an athlete can adapt to a an increasing stress load in the form of training stimuli...When an organism is in a situation where its physiology is functioning at optimal levels with the least amount of energy expenditure it is considered to be in a state of stasis... "* -Bob Takano[4]

Takano compares training within confines to training beyond threshold and how it can disrupt homeostasis. I am going to analogize his example here: If an athlete regularly consumes a certain amount of calories for a certain number of days and weeks to maintain their body, and begins to increase training volume slightly over time, the body will adapt to the additional training demands without increasing its energy demands. This gradual rise of volume and the subsequent adaptation of the tissues qualifies this as a eustress, or good stress.[5] If the same athlete were to decrease calories on the same training program, the athlete may reach a point where they cannot recover sufficiently between training sessions, and may become more susceptible to injury or illness. Thus, the hypocaloric diet is considered a distress, or bad stress. Unneeded stress is the last thing an athlete needs to add to his/her plate.

Fortunately, your lifestyle multiplier will account for this stress. However, if your training intensifies, you may need to raise your multiplier (or lower it, if your training decreases). I previously noted that your multiplier is not

4,-   Tanako, Bob. *Homeostasis: The Basis of Training* [Internet] 2013 Nov 5. Catalyst Athletics. http://www.catalystathletics.com/article/1810/Homeostasis-The-Basis-of-Training/

5   http://www.takanoathletics.com/

a permanent number and will likely change as your training and goals do, especially if you are a competitive or professional athlete (in-season training and nutrition will look different than it does in the off-season).

It is important for competitive athletes to remain in a state of homeostasis for several reasons:

- The importance of physical exercise in regulating energy balance and body mass is widely recognized.[6]
- From all nutritional variables, optimal energy supply is considered most vital for human performance. It is postulated that lack of energy homeostasis is the basic problem in the development of overtraining.[7]
- Change is stressful on your body. Adding (or losing) tissue forces your body to recalibrate itself to a new weight. If your body is regularly subjected to the stress of gaining or losing weight, it will perform better with the weight fluctuation variable removed.
- Homeostasis creates an internal equilibrium in spite of external day-to-day factors that affect us (eg: break-ups, school, work). Being in a state of homeostasis is low stress, which makes it easier to deal with unexpected circumstances in life.
- The systems of our body and our organs thrive in [homeostasis].[8] If any part of the nervous system is damaged, homeostasis is difficult or impossible to maintain.[9]

6   Jürimäe J, Mäestu J, Jürimäe T, Mangus B, von Duvillard SP, authors. Peripheral signals of energy homeostasis as possible markers of training stress in athletes: a review. Metabolism. 2011 Mar 60(3):335-50. doi: 10.1016. Accessed at: http://www.ncbi.nlm.nih.gov/pubmed/20304442

7   Saris WH, author. The concept of energy homeostasis for optimal health during training. Can J Appl Physiol. 2001;26 Suppl:S167-75. Accessed at: http://www.ncbi.nlm.nih.gov/pubmed/11897892

8   McGraw Hill College Division. Body Systems and Homeostasis. 1997. Accessed 2015 January 15 at: http://www.mhhe.com/biosci/genbio/maderbiology/supp/homeo.html

9   WiseGEEK. What Is the Connection Between the Nervous System and Homeostasis? [Internet] Accessed 5 January 2015 at: http://www.wisegeekhealth.com/what-is-the-connection-between-the-nervous-system-and-homeostasis.htm

But athletes are not the only population that are encouraged to eat at maintenance. Included are those individuals who want to remain at the same weight, but improve overall body composition. For example, a woman who is 5'4", weighs 120 pounds, and has 27% body fat doesn't need to lose *weight*, per se. Rather, she should aim to lower her body fat percentage while maintaining weight, with the result being an accompanying increase in relative lean body mass. This example of what is commonly referred to as "skinny fat" is applicable to men, too. A 6'0 tall man weighing 200 pounds sounds like a stud, but a man who is 10% body fat is going to look drastically different than a man who is 25% body fat at that weight. The latter should prioritize fat tissue loss above pure weight loss.

If your training is on point, there is no reason to think that your body won't change. If you are doing enough volume and a sufficient amount of conditioning (note I said conditioning and not cardio… so shameless plug: Black Iron's MET[abolic]CON[ditioning]), you will see physical changes, assuming you are eating enough to repair the tissue damage you are incurring with regular training.

I know what you are thinking: *Can I gain muscle and lose fat at the same time?* This is the Holy Grail of performance and nutrition, and the answer is as sought after as the Ark of the Covenant (shout out to Dr. Jones). The truth is, there isn't a definitive yes or no answer to this question. If taken literally, the answer is no. From a physiological standpoint you cannot put on muscle and burn fat at exactly the same time (anabolism and catabolism are exclusive states). But over a long period of time, it is possible, although not easy to do. It takes extreme dedication to both your eating and your training. Eating at maintenance is more ideally suited to this situation because your caloric intake is low enough to avoid weight gain, but high enough to support the development of new muscle tissue. By eating at maintenance rather than a caloric surplus, you will lose fat quicker than you will gain muscle. In all likelihood, you won't lose 15 pounds of fat and put on 15 pounds of muscle in 12 weeks time. But, it is not unreasonable to lose 10 pounds of fat and put on 5 pounds of muscle in 12 weeks time, which would have a dramatic affect on how your body looked. Keep in mind that if you are taking the body recomp route via eating at maintenance, it isn't a fast process. Patience you must have, young Padawan.

There are countess articles you can read online with a simple Google search if this subject interests you further. The most important thing to remember is that you must be weight training daily, and you must be conditioning daily if you choose to seek out the Holy Grail.

Long Story Short...

- If you are an athlete with a multiplier between 14-16 and are getting ready for a competition that doesn't require you to drop weight (to make a weight class, for instance) , you should be eating at maintenance.
- If you are a healthy weight for you height, but want to undergo a modest recomposition, you should be eating at maintenance coupled with an intense training program. (Note: if you want to lose more than 5% BF or 15 pounds, your primary goal should switch to weight loss for a few months).
- If you are in no rush for dramatic changes in either direction (weight loss or gain), and simply want to enjoy flexible dieting, you should be eating at maintenance.

Sources & Further Reading Suggestions:

Jürimäe, Jaak et al., authors. Peripheral signals of energy homeostasis as possible markers of training stress in athletes: a review. Metabolism - Clinical and Experimental, Volume 60 , Issue 3 , 335 - 350. Accessed at:
 http://www.sciencedirect.com/science/article/pii/S0026049510000636

Clemens Drenowatz, Joey C. Eisenmann, Joseph J. Carlson, Karin A. Pfeiffer, James M. Pivarnik, authors. Energy expenditure and dietary intake during high-volume and low-volume training periods among male endurance athletes. Applied Physiology, Nutrition, and Metabolism, 2012, 37(2): 199-205, 10.1139/h11-155 Accessed at: http://www.nrcresearchpress.com/doi/abs/10.1139/h2001-051#. VNGQSGTF92c

Saris WH, author. The concept of energy homeostasis for optimal health during training. Can J Appl Physiol. 2001;26 Suppl:S167-75. Accessed at:
http://www.ncbi.nlm.nih.gov/pubmed/11897892

WiseGEEK. What Is the Connection Between the Nervous System and Homeostasis? [Internet] Accessed 5 January 2015 at: http://www.wisegeekhealth.com/what-is-the-connection-between-the-nervous-system-and-homeostasis.htm

McGraw-Hill College Division. Body Systems and Homeostasis. Accessed at:
http://www.mhhe.com/biosci/genbio/maderbiology/supp/homeo.html

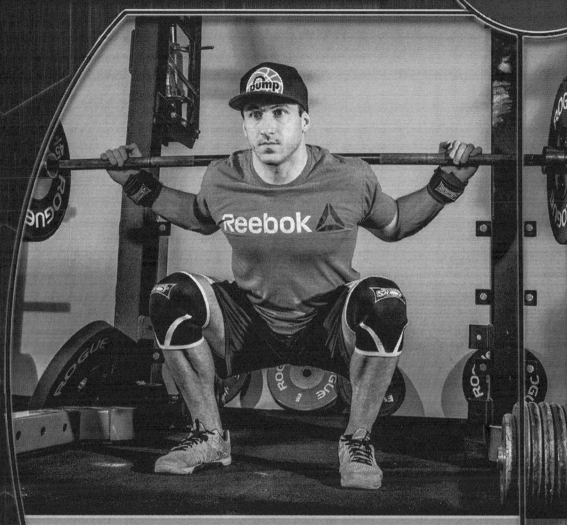

"SILENT MIKE" FARR
POWERLIFTING

"SILENT MIKE" FARR

WHO ARE YOU AND WHAT DO YOU DO?

MY NAME IS "SILENT MIKE" FARR. I AM A COACH AND POWERLIFTER FROM NORTHERN CALIFORNIA.

WHAT IS YOUR PERSONAL DEFINITION OF FLEXIBLE DIETING?

FLEXIBLE DIETING IS A WAY OF EATING THAT ENABLES ATHLETES TO BE IN FULL CONTROL AND STAY CONSISTENT 24/7- 365 WHILE HAVING A "NORMAL" LIFE. FOR ME, FLEXIBLE DIETING IS A SIMPLE STRATEGY THAT TAUGHT ME MODERATION AND BALANCE ALL THE WHILE ALLOWING FREEDOM IN MY FOOD CHOICES.

WHEN DID YOU START FLEXIBLE DIETING?

I BEGAN FLEXIBLE DIETING NEARLY 3 YEARS AGO AFTER READING AND RESEARCHING THOSE THAT HAVE USED IT IN THE COMPETITIVE STRENGTH WORLD.

WHAT WAS YOUR DIET LIKE BEFORE FLEXIBLE DIETING?

BEFORE FLEXIBLE DIETING I HAD TRIED MANY DIFFERENT TYPES OF NUTRITIONAL STRATEGIES BUT COULD NEVER STAY CONSISTENT. AS A STRENGTH ATHLETE, I ALWAYS PUT A PRIORITY ON PROTEIN BUT AFTER THAT I WOULD EAT NEARLY ANYTHING I WANTED. I WENT THROUGH A LOW CARB PHASE BUT NEVER COULD GET THE RESULTS OF BEING LEAN AND GAINING THE STRENGTH THAT I DESIRED.

WHAT HAVE BEEN YOUR BIGGEST STRENGTH BREAKTHROUGHS IN EACH SINCE SWITCHING TO FLEXIBLE DIETING? WHAT ABOUT AESTHETIC BREAKTHROUGHS?

RECENTLY, WITHIN THE LAST YEAR, I DECIDED TO GO ON A CUT, MOSTLY TO LOOK BETTER BUT ALSO TO BE A LITTLE CLOSER TO MY COMPETING WEIGHT CLASS. THROUGH FLEXIBLE DIETING, I DECIDED TO DO A NICE SLOW CUT, TRYING TO HOLD ON TO AS MUCH STRENGTH AS I COULD. WHILE DROPPING AROUND 20 LBS, I WAS ABLE TO KEEP NEARLY ALL MY STRENGTH AND NEVER ONCE FELT LIKE I WAS DIETING. I WAS NEVER TIRED, FATIGUED OR STARVING. SINCE THEN, I HAVE UPPED MY CALORIES A BIT AND AM SLOWLY GAINING WEIGHT BACK. THE ACCURACY AND CONSISTENCY OF FLEXIBLE DIETING HAS ALLOWED ME TO STAY LEAN WHILE GET ENOUGH CALORIES TO CONTINUE TO GROW AND GET STRONGER.

WHAT ARE YOUR THREE MOST IMPORTANT GUIDELINES YOU GIVE YOURSELF IN REGARD TO NUTRITION?

1. HIT MY DAILY MACRO-NUTRIENT GOALS.
2. FOCUS ON MICRO-NUTRIENT DENSE FOODS.
3. ALLOW MYSELF TO EAT (IN MODERATION) THE FOODS I LIKE OR CRAVE.

"SILENT MIKE" FARR

WHAT IS THE BEST PIECE OF ADVICE YOU WISH YOU HAD AT THE START OF YOUR JOURNEY THAT COULD HELP NEWBIES?

ALTHOUGHT FLEXIBLE DIETING IS AN EASY STRATEGY FOR EVERYONE, TRACKING YOUR FOODS CONSISTENTLY AND ACCURATELY IS A SKILL. HITTING YOUR DAILY MACRO-NUTRIENT REQUIREMENTS AND TRACKING EVERYTHING YOU EAT IS IMPERATIVE FOR YOU TO REACH YOUR GOALS. THERE WILL BE UPS AND DOWNS IN YOUR PROGRESS BUT THE NUMBER ONE THING IS ALWAYS CONSISTENCY.

ADDITIONAL COMMENTS:

I WANT TO THANK KRISSY FOR REACHING OUT AND HAVING ME BE A PART OF THIS PROJECT. IF YOU GUYS ARE INTERESTED IN LEARNING MORE ABOUT WHAT I DO, YOU CAN CHECKOUT WWW.SUPERTRAINING.TV OR MARK BELL'S POWERCAST ON ITUNES.

7. Eating At A Caloric Deficit (Cutting)

There are many reasons why someone would want to lose weight. Regardless if you're losing weight to make a weight class, get better at gymnastic movements, or simply want to look better naked, the science remains the same: fewer calories must be consumed than being used in order for the body to be coerced into recruiting stored tissue for energy. Again, *tissue*, meaning fat and muscle. By consuming fewer calories than you're burning, the body is put into a negative balance and mass will always be lost. Simply put, in order to lose weight one must lower caloric intake **OR**, increase activity level so that more calories are burned than are being taken in (I suggest a combination of the two), and over the course of several weeks or months, this will result in weight loss.

The goal with eating at a deficit should *always* be **to eat as much as possible while still losing weight**. A sizable deficit is often not only unnecessary, but dangerous, too, and will have negative long-term effects on the systems of the body. Too many people want to take short cuts to get weight off, which brings me to a very cliché statement: "you didn't put the weight on overnight, you're not going to get it off overnight, either". If you want a diet that will get weight off quick, you bought the wrong book, dawg. The slow approach is the best approach if you are seeking **maintainable** fat loss as there should be no end goal of "leanness". Let's say you achieve an impressive level of leanness, then what? Do you scream, "I am fitness!" from the rooftops and retire? No. You should seek more of a long-term sustainable combination of leanness, athleticism, and overall well-being that is maintainable without making you miserable.

By now you've determined your maintenance calories, which means that you have a fairly solid starting position as far as a "cut" is concerned. If you heeded the earlier advice of verifying your maintenance for two weeks, you are in an even *more* advantageous position. Now it's time to determine your optimal caloric deficit so as to better help you achieve your individual weight loss goals.

Determining Your Deficit

First and foremost, any weight loss above 1-2 pounds a week is likely at the expense of hard muscle tissue, as well, at a roughly 1:1 ratio to fat. Prevailing wisdom when it comes to weight loss is that an accumulated 3500 kcal deficit is required per pound of tissue loss.[10] This means that a 3500-7000 weekly caloric deficit would do the trick of facilitating a 1-2 pound weekly drop. Too many people think that this automatically means to cut that many calories a week, ignoring the fact that physical activity is a potent part of the equation. This is where you need to ask yourself the following question: "Can I make the time to train an extra 10-20 minutes a day?" and I am hoping you figure out a way to enthusiastically say, "HELL YES!"

---

10   Hall KD, author. Body fat and fat-free mass inter-relationships: Forbes's theory revisited [Internet]. Br J Nutr. 2007 Jun;97(6):1059-63. Epub 2007 Mar 19. Accessed at http://www.ncbi. nlm.nih.gov/pubmed/17367567.

Why, for example, would you cut 500 calories per day when you would only have to cut 250? Between 10 minutes of intense conditioning and the subsequent *excess post-exercise oxygen consumption (EPOC)*, also known as *afterburn*, you'll be at your desired deficit and subsequently be able to eat more. "EPOC is accompanied by an elevated consumption of fuel. In response to exercise, fat stores are broken down and free fatty acids (FFAs) are released into the bloodstream. In recovery, the direct oxidation of free fatty acids as fuel and the energy consuming re-conversion of FFAs back into fat stores both take place."[11] If you train at an intense enough pace, EPOC can be responsible for creating a larger deficit than you would have achieved if you skipped training and lowered calories.

I am a huge advocate of "eat more, train more" as opposed to "cut all the calories and feel sluggish during workouts". Those extra 250 calories could end up giving you the boost to complete a 20 minute conditioning piece that, through improved EPOC, may end up putting you at a larger deficit than you would have achieved if you had opted to eat less, instead.

Cutting anywhere from 100-1000 calories a day, or 700-7000 calories over the course of a week, will lead to weight loss. That is a large range, but I want to show how arbitrary it is to say you should "lower daily caloric intake by 500", since that won't work for every person who is attempting to lose weight. Given that our bodies and goals are unique, the caloric deficits we choose for ourselves should be equally unique. Many factors, like age and weight, affect the rate at which both genders lose weight, and some people drop weight much easier than others. If an overweight woman with an estimated maintenance of 2900 calories per day cuts her daily caloric intake by the oft-recommended 500 calories, she's still at a fairly high caloric intake of 2400 calories a day, and has significant room to safely cut much more. In comparison, if a lighter female with a maintenance intake of 1800 calories were to subtract the same 500 calories from her diet, she'd be eating 1300 calories a day, which isn't

---

11 Excess Post-Exercise Oxygen Consumption. Accessed 5 January 2015 at http://en.wikipedia.org/wiki/Excess_post-exercise_oxygen_consumption

much food, and leaves with her with very little caloric "wiggle-room" if and when she plateaus. There are obvious problems with generic, "one size fits all" calorie reduction as it produces largely different outcomes in each person.

This is yet another reason to be in-tune with your body and experiment with yourself. To use myself as an example, I know that if I were to cut 600 calories a day, I could expect to lose two or more pounds by the end of the week, but I also know that I need a deficit larger than 200 calories to lose any weight. This is something I have learned about myself over years of dedicated practice and experimentation. I didn't learn it overnight; it took a lot of trial and error, patience, and consistency.

IMPORTANT: if you have a lot of weight to get off, you can get away with a larger deficit. If you are already small or lean, you won't need a large deficit as there isn't as much to lose. Your maintenance calories will demonstrate this.

To put it simply, it is better to leave yourself some wiggle room than it is to cut too much, too soon, and have nowhere left to go. I suggest doing the following: start with a 300-600 calorie deficit, preferably from a combination of eating less and training more (remember our discussion on EPOC). You can choose to break it up however you please, but if you are losing weight too quickly (more that 2 pounds a week), add 100 calories a day back into your diet. Conversely, if you don't see weight loss results in a few weeks' time, try lowering your daily intake 100 calories, and see where you're at in another couple weeks. If you are making **zero** progress after repeatedly lowering your calories, and find yourself approaching a 1000 calorie deficit, it is in your best interest to hire a coach to assist you in your efforts. Coaches can be beneficial for two reasons: they can (1) hold you more accountable, which will ensure consistency when you may otherwise be a little too lenient, and they can help you (2) pinpoint what you have been doing wrong, and give you a more accurate calculation.

There are a few exceptions that would make someone exempt from the

"1-2 pounds a week" rule of thumb.

> *"Both research and practical experience have shown that the optimal rates of tissue change seem to be supported by a 1-2 lbs (0.5-1.0kg) per week weight loss or gain. These numbers apply to most individuals under most circumstances. Exotic situations and individuals (those weighing below 100 lbs and far in excess of 300 lbs, for example) may call for different recommendations, to be discussed with a body composition diet coach. "* -The Renaissance Diet, by Nick Shaw and Mike Israetel

If You Have A Lot Of Weight To Lose...

Someone who has between 50-100 (or even more) pounds to lose should be treated a bit differently, as the maintenance calculation may be overwhelmingly high. If you, or your client, are substantially overweight, I would avoid calculating a deficit and instead do the following: set multiple short-term, *realistic* weight loss goals in 8-12 week increments and calculate caloric maintenance for each goal by selecting the appropriate multiplier for the individual. For example, a 250 pound woman may have an initial short-term weight loss goal to reach 225 pounds; a mid-term goal to reach 200 pounds; and a long-term goal to reach 180 pounds. A person could reasonably drop 70-80 pounds in 24-36 weeks (extremely overweight people can safely lose 3-4 pounds a week). Once each goal weight has been achieved, eat at maintenance for the next goal weight, so on. However, once someone has lost a lot of weight on the scale, they should stop using the scale as their primary measure of progress. Once you've reached a healthy, comfortable weight, you can switch over to eating at a deficit for you current weight as described at the beginning of this chapter.

If You Are Already Fairly Lean...

If you are already fairly lean, you are going to have a harder time losing fat. If you have a low body fat and you want it lower, it is safe to assume that your goals are strictly aesthetic at this point (which is fine). You will need a very small deficit of 100-300 calories a day, which will likely equate to a slower rate of weight loss, perhaps only ½ pound a week. Aesthetic goals require far more accuracy in tracking, which we will discuss in Chapter 9. Lastly, if your metabolism is not in good standing and you have been under-eating for months, you will have a hell of a time trying to shed more weight from an already lean physique. I suggest eating at maintenance for a few weeks, but continuing to train hard so as to give your body a break from a prolonged hypocaloric state, especially if you find that you've hit a stubborn plateau.

Plateauing While On A Cut...

Here's a nugget of truth: it is inevitable at some point during a cut that you will begin to plateau. If you achieve your goal before hitting a plateau, you are a very special, and fortunate case (high five!). If you are not one of the very lucky ones, you need to be prepared and know what to do when a plateau hits. Plateaus typically hit because your body is no longer in homeostasis and the stress of training and dieting have caught up to you. You can slowly cut more calories or you can add a few conditioning sessions, but eventually you will hit a wall.

Your body kind of says, "no more" one day because it has been pulled in opposite directions for too long… you kept training more and you kept eating less. The human body has evolved and adapted since the dawn of man and it is designed to survive. This is your body surviving.

At this point in time, you have a few options:

1. If you have lost weight (whether it be 5 pounds or 30 pounds), recalculate

your calories based off your new weight. Something to consider, is that if you intensified training past your original multiplier to get weight off, you may want to use a higher multiplier. From here you can calculate maintenance then determine a new deficit.

2. If your cut was working well and then started to slow down, and you refuse to lower calories, you should take take a deload training week and introduce some more calories into your diet for a week to give your body a quick break, then continue doing what you were doing.

3. If you are not losing any weight at all, you should think about eating at maintenance for a month and being extremely consistent as your body is giving you every signal it can that it isn't ready to lose weight yet. You may need to get your metabolism back in good standing.

Lastly, if your cut is moving along with no issues and you continue to see healthy and gratifying results, don't ask anyone when you should recalculate or do something different. To quote Jesus Christ, "Don't fix what isn't broken" (I think that's who said it, but it's been awhile since shop class).

A Few Thoughts On The Scale

If you are more comfortable staying off of it (which I highly suggest for most people, especially women), please do. If you find the number isn't decreasing, don't think that progress isn't being made. Remember what I said at the beginning of the book in regard to setting physical goals, as well? You look at yourself in the mirror every single day so sometimes it is hard to see physical changes, but don't rely on the slab of glass in your bathroom to be the judge. Take measurements and progress pictures instead, as these will give you equally verifiable (and less variable) measures of your progress, whereas the number on the scale is subject to change on a daily, even hourly, basis. For me, the best affirmation of my progress is the progress I make in the gym. I have battled body dysmorphia since I was a teenager, and where I used to seek validation from the scale, I now seek validation from a barbell. This has been one of the best things I have ever done for mys

When You Should Care About The Scale: Making Weight

On the flip side, if you need to make weight for your sport you need to be on the scale. Competitive athletes tend to have an easier time weighing themselves since they are more performance-oriented, rather than aesthetically-driven. If you are attempting to make weight, I recommend the following:

1. Count how many weeks you have from now until your weigh-in.

2. Divide how many pounds you have to lose into those weeks to determine the slowest and most consistent way to lose weight.

3. Determine an appropriate calorie cut based off how many pounds a week you need to lose in order to make weight.

Example time: If you have a meet in 12 weeks, and you need to drop 8 pounds to make your desired weight class, you should aim to lose 0.67 pounds per week, which is approximately a 2,345 weekly caloric deficit.

desired weight loss in lbs ÷ wks to achieve goal = lbs lost per wk x 3500 = wkly deficit

The slow approach is the right approach in every situation, especially for athletes. If you lose too much weight too soon, your performance will inevitably suffer. With that being said, once you establish an effective caloric deficit, you can optimize your fat loss by appropriately distributing the proper amount of protein, carbs, and fat in order to get the best results possible, which we will cover in Chapter Nine.

Sources & Further Reading Suggestions:

Hall KD., author. Body fat and fat-free mass inter-relationships: Forbes's theory revisited. Br J Nutr. 2007 Jun;97(6):1059-63. Epub 2007 Mar 19. Accessed at:
http://www.ncbi.nlm.nih.gov/pubmed/17367567

Hall KD., author. What is the required energy deficit per unit weight loss? Int J Obes (Lond). 2008 Mar;32(3):573-6. Epub 2007 Sep 11.
Accessed at: http://www.ncbi.nlm.nih.gov/pubmed/17848938

Stiegler P, Cunliffe A, authors. The role of diet and exercise for the maintenance of fat-free mass and resting metabolic rate during weight loss. Sports Med. 2006;36(3):239-62. Accessed at:
http://www.ncbi.nlm.nih.gov/pubmed/16526835

Van Gaal LF, Vansant GA, De Leeuw IH., authors. Factors determining energy expenditure during very-low-calorie diets. Am J Clin Nutr. 1992 Jul;56(1 Suppl):224S-229S. Accessed at:
http://www.ncbi.nlm.nih.gov/pubmed/1615888

Dr. Jade Tada, author. EPOC Exposed: Why It Can't Completely Explain the Metabolic Afterburn. Metabolic Effect. Accessed at:
http://www.metaboliceffect.com/epoc-exposed-why-it-cant-completely-explain-the-metabolic-after-burn/

Rena R Wing and Suzanne Phelan, authors. Long-term weight loss maintenance.
The American Journal of Clinical Nutrition. American Society for Clinical Nutrition. 2005. Accessed at:
http://ajcn.nutrition.org/content/82/1/222S.long

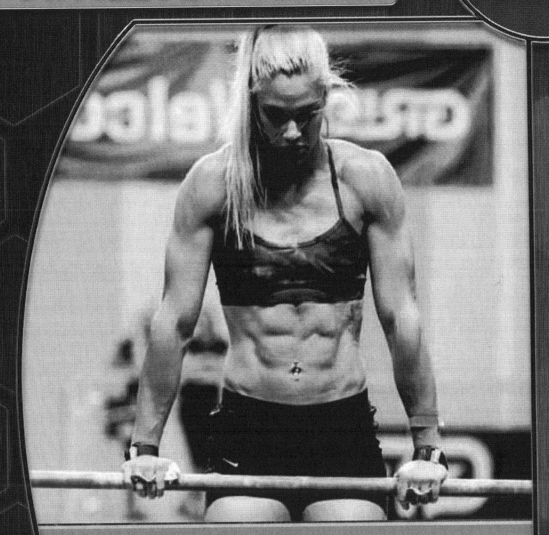

ATHLETE PROFILE

NICOLE CAPRUSO
CROSSFIT/NPGL ATHLETE

NICOLE CAPRUSO

WHO ARE YOU AND WHAT DO YOU DO?

I AM A FORMER DIVISION 1 BASKETBALL PLAYER AT HOFSTRA UNIVERSITY IN LONG ISLAND, NY. I GRADUATED FROM HOFSTRA IN 2012 WITH A BS IN EXERCISE SCIENCE. I AM A CERTIFIED PERSONAL TRAINER UNDER NCSF, HAVE A SPORTS NUTRITION CERTIFICATION WITH THEM AS WELL AS A PRE AND POST NATAL TRAINING CERTIFICATION. I AM CFL1 CERTIFIED AS WELL AS USAW L1 CERTIFIED. ABOUT A YEAR OR SO AFTER GRADUATION AND NO LONGER BEING COMPETITIVE IN SPORTS, I REALIZED I MISSED IT TREMENDOUSLY! I THEN FOUND CROSSFIT, AND SHORTLY AFTER THAT WEIGHTLIFTING. I NOW MANAGE A GYM WHERE I COACH MOST OF THE CROSSFIT CLASSES. I ALSO RUN A FLEXIBLE DIETING COACHING BUSINESS WHERE I GUIDE CLIENTS ON HOW TO USE FLEXIBLE DIETING TO REACH THEIR GOALS, BOTH PHYSICALLY AND ATHLETICALLY.

WHEN DID YOU START FLEXIBLE DIETING AND WHY?

IN MAY OF 2014 I BEGAN FLEXIBLE DIETING. I NEEDED TO CUT WEIGHT FOR USAW NATIONALS THAT WAS TAKING PLACE IN JULY OF 2014. I WAS WALKING AROUND AT PROBABLY THE HEAVIEST I HAD EVER BEEN AND I KNEW I WOULD NEED A GREAT COACH AND PROGRAM TO GET ME TO BE ABLE TO COMPETE IN MY DESIRED WEIGHT CLASS. I REACHED OUT TO RICKLYNN LONG AND SHE STARTED ME ON A PROGRAM TO REVAMP MY METABOLISM AND HELP ME CUT WEIGHT SAFELY AND HAPPILY.

WHAT WAS YOUR DIET LIKE BEFORE FLEXIBLE DIETING?

MY ENTIRE LIFE I NEVER WORRIED ABOUT FOOD, WHAT I ATE, OR WHAT I WEIGHED. I JUST DIDN'T NEED TO. WHEN I STARTED WEIGHTLIFTING AND HAVING TO "MAKE WEIGHT" AT MEETS WAS MY FIRST INTERACTION WITH GETTING ON A SCALE. IN DECEMBER OF 2013 I CUT WEIGHT FOR THE AMERICAN OPEN USING A VERY STRICT, TUPPERWARE CRASH DIET – LIKELY CONSUMING UNDER 1000 CALORIES PER DAY. I LOST WEIGHT AND MADE WEIGHT FOR THE MEET, BUT I SEVERELY DAMAGED MY BODY AND MY METABOLISM IN THE PROCESS. AFTER THAT, I WENT BACK TO EATING 80/20 PALEO THINKING THAT WAS THE ANSWER AND IT JUST WAS NOT THE CASE. I WAS TRAINING VIGOROUSLY FOR REGIONALS AND EATING AS CLEAN AS I COULD TOLERATE YET WAS STILL PACKING ON WEIGHT. BY THE TIME I REACHED OUT TO RICKLYNN, I WAS ABOUT 8KG HEAVIER THAN I HAD BEEN ONLY A FEW MONTHS PRIOR. THAT IS WHEN I FOUND FD AND SAW THE LIGHT!

WHAT WAS IT LIKE CUTTING WEIGHT FOR A MEET BUT MAINTAINING STRENGTH THROUGH FLEXIBLE DIETING?

THE GAME CHANGER FOR ME (AND THE MINUTE I WAS SOLD) WAS WHEN I DROPPED ABOUT 3KG WITHIN THE FIRST 10DAYS OF FLEXIBLE DIETING AS WELL AS HITTING EIGHT, YES EIGHT PR'S THAT SAME WEEK. I REALIZED THAT MY BODY WAS MUCH MORE COMFORTABLE WITH THE INTRODUCTION OF MORE CARBS AND ALSO WITH THE OVERALL BALANCE FLEXIBLE DIETING PROVIDED. EVEN IN THE DEPTHS OF MY INITIAL CUT WHEN I WAS EATING UNDER 1600 CALORIES A DAY, I WAS STILL HITTING HUGE LIGHTS AND MAINTAINING STRENGTH NUMBERS THAT I HAD AT A BODYWEIGHT ABOUT 6KG HEAVIER. I LEARNED WHERE TO PLACE CERTAIN MACROS AROUND MY WORKOUT TO MAKE ME FEEL GREAT IN THE GYM EVEN ON A LIMITED CALORIC INTAKE. I HAVE CUT WEIGHT TWO WAYS. ONE INVOLVED A CRASH DIET AND CARRYING A TUPPAWARE ALL OVER. THIS RESULTED IN A VERY WEAK, HUNGRY, AND NOT VERY MUSCULAR ATHLETE. THE BETTER OPTION INVOLVED BEING ABLE TO EAT ANYTHING IN THE CORRECT PROPORTIONS, EVEN IF THAT ONLY MEANT HALF OF A DOUGHNUT, A LONG LIST OF PR'S ALONG THE

WAY, AND THE LOWEST BODY FAT I HAVE EVER SEEN WITH A SIGNIFICANT INCREASE IN MUSCLE MASS.

WHAT HAS BEEN YOUR BIGGEST BREAKTHROUGH SINCE FLEXIBLE DIETING?

THE BIGGEST BREAKTHROUGH WITH ME FOR FLEXIBLE DIETING HAS BEEN THE WAY I NOW EQUATE FOOD WITH ENERGY AND THE MEANS TO FUEL ME AS AN ATHLETE. WHILE TRYING TO FOLLOW A "CLEAN EATING" OR "PALEO" STYLE DIET I WAS ALWAYS CONCERNED THAT IF I ATE A FORBIDDEN FOOD, OR HAD A "CHEAT MEAL" NO MATTER HOW SMALL, IT WAS GOING TO HAVE A NEGATIVE EFFECT ON ME AS AN ATHLETE AND I WAS SOMEHOW GOING TO BE WORSE IN THE GYM BECAUSE OF IT. IT WOULD MAKE ME FEEL GUILTY OR BAD AND MAKE ME THINK I WAS A TERRIBLY DEDICATED ATHLETE FOR HAVING ONE MEASLY CHOCOLATE CHIP COOKIE! I NOW HAVE LEARNED THAT BALANCE IS THE KEY TO ATHLETIC SUCCESS, AND THE JOYS OF LIFE NEED TO BE INCORPORATED IN THERE – MOST IMPORTANTLY IN ORDER TO FUEL YOU AS AN ATHLETE!

WHAT IS THE BEST PIECE OF ADVICE YOU WISH YOU HAD WHEN STARTING FLEXIBLE DIETING THAT COULD HELP NEWBIES?

DO YOUR RESEARCH AND UNDERSTAND THE SCIENCE BEHIND WHAT YOU ARE DOING. DO NOT RELY ON A COACH TO JUST GIVE YOU NUMBERS AND TELL YOU TO FOLLOW THEM. ASK QUESTIONS, UNDERSTAND THE PROCESS, LEARN ABOUT YOUR BODY AND STAY IN TUNE WITH HOW YOU FEEL. UNDERSTAND THINGS LIKE "REFEED" DAYS ARE CAREFULLY CALCULATED, NOT FREE FOR ALLS; REVERSE DIETS ARE THE GOLDEN GIFT TO FLEXIBLE DIETING, SO WHETHER THE STORM OF A HARD CUT, AND MOST IMPORTANTLY, VIEW YOUR DEDICATION TO YOUR FOOD PROGRAM THE SAME WAY YOU VIEW YOUR DEDICATION TO YOUR FITNESS PROGRAM… THEY ARE ONE IN THE SAME!

8. Eating At A Caloric Surplus

This chapter won't be as dense as the previous one. Gaining weight tends to be a more enjoyable, and simpler, process than losing it, since you won't need to be nearly as accurate or stringent with your diet. As quoted by Shaw and Israetel in the previous chapter, weight gain exceeding 2lbs per week is likely the bad kind of weight that you will eventually want off. Just as with weight loss, 1-2lbs a week is the best route to maximize muscular development and minimal fat growth. Now there are two types of #gainz, the visible, aesthetic kind, and the physical strength kind.

Visible Gains

There are several reasons why someone may want to gain weight. Whether you are recovering from an eating disorder, are on a journey to real manhood (which refers to a male weighing more than 200 pounds), or you want to be the swolest bro (or she-bro) at your local globo-gym, you need to be eating more calories than you are burning.

We already know that a 3500-7000 calorie-a-week influx from maintenance will yield 1-2 pounds of tissue gain, so eat up, champ. If you struggle with gaining weight, you may need to eat more, which is perfectly fine. If you have a lot of weight to gain, you can go above the recommended 500-1000 daily caloric surplus. However, some people struggle with weight gain because they don't know *what* to eat, which we will discuss in later chapters.

Furthermore, when eating at a surplus for hypertrophy, your training needs to be heavy and high volume. High volume = muscular hypertrophy, and a caloric surplus will facilitate this hypertrophy.

What To Do If You Stop Gaining Weight

Some people hit weight gain plateaus. Treat these the same as you would a weight loss plateau:

1. If you have gained weight (whether it be 5 pounds or 30 pounds), recalculate your calories based off of your new body weight and proper multiplier. From here you can re-approach the entire process from a fresh start.

2. If your bulk was working well and then started to slow down, and you can't stuff your mouth hole with anymore food, you should go back to maintenance for a week or two and take a deload week from training to give your body a quick break from metabolizing a metric fuck ton of food, then resume your normal training and diet regimen.

3. If you are not gaining any weight at all, you should consider eating at maintenance consistently for a month, as your body may be giving you signals that is not yet ready for all the #gainz quite yet.

Physical Gains

In Chapter Six we discussed a eucaloric diet being optimal for most elite athletes. This isn't the case for a novice lifter looking to make serious strength gains. If an intense new program is introduced to a novice lifter or athlete, the body is going to need the appropriate nutritional approach for progress to be made. Let's take an underdeveloped (this is a nice way of saying "skinny") male who has minimal lifting experience and weighs 160lbs. Said gentleman wants to put 100 pounds on each of the three main lifts: squat, bench, and deadlift. The programming for this will likely be a lot for this young man to handle and, for the sake of recovery, mass, and power, his diet should be hypercaloric until he reaches his stated strength goals. The primary goal is increased performance and any accompanying weight gain will be a byproduct of the training and the surplus.

Since there is usually no body weight goal attached to non-competitive strength and performance goals, the dieter does not need to eat at a specific calculated surplus, nor do they need to step on a scale. Simply going above maintenance and eating when hungry should suffice for strength enhancement. Protein requirement should be calculated and met daily, but beyond that it turns into a loose "eat more carbs if you aren't getting stronger" suggestion. Once the athlete is no longer a "novice", he or she can reapproach flexible dieting from the beginning to achieve whatever desired goal they've since adopted. The programming and dieting will both evolve with the athlete.

By now you should have decided if your goal is to maintain, cut, or gain weight, as well as determined how many calories you will be consuming daily to reach your goal, which means more fun math is required! Pencils and Scantrons ready?

SO YOU'RE AT HOME AND YOU WANT TO TAKE A TRIP

WHERE DO YOU WANT TO GO?

TAKE THE ROAD TO
SHRED CITY

TAKE THE GAIN TRAIN
TO GAINZVILLE

YOUR JOURNEY IS GOING FINE
UNTIL YOU END UP AT THE PLATEAU

WHAT DO YOU NEED TO DO
TO GET BACK ON TRACK?

RECALCULATE
YOUR MACROS

EAT AT MAINTENCE
FOR A FEW WEEKS

DELOAD WEEK
FOR MORE CALS

DELOAD WEEK
FOR FEWER CALS

AND NOW YOU ARE THERE

AND NOW YOU ARE THERE

9. Calculating & Optimizing Your Macros

Second to calorie balance, macronutrients are the next important component for optimizing flexible dieting. We went over protein, carbs, and fat in detail in Chapter Four and we can put that information to use now provided you have your daily caloric intake figured out (or, at least have a starting place). Like every other aspect of your life, structure is important. You have to put a plan in motion to get the most out of this. This goes beyond just counting calories, as you need to optimize which macros will yield a certain amount of the *right* calories.

There is one more thing that I want to make **very** clear before we start calculating macros. The numbers you are about to come up with are simply an *estimate*, the purpose of which is to give you an *approximate* starting point. This will suffice to get you started, but you may find that you need to make some tweaks and adjustments to really dial this in. We are first going to calculate your starting point before discussing in greater detail how to optimize your macro profile later in the chapter.

First, convert your body weight from pounds to kilograms. This is very easy to do with the calculator on your smartphone. Divide your body weight by 2.2 to get your weight in kilos:

body weight in pounds ÷ 2.2 = body weight in kilograms

Protein is calculated first as it is the superior macronutrient. Protein supports muscle growth, thus is takes precedence. We want 2g of protein per kilogram of bodyweight. Take your weight in kilos and multiply it by 2 to determine how many grams of protein you should consume a day. Each gram of protein is going to be responsible for 4 calories of your total daily caloric intake.

body weight in kilograms x 2 = grams of protein per day

grams of protein per day x 4 (cals/gram) = daily calories from protein

Fat is calculated second as it makes calculating your carbs easier by doing it in this order. This is a major yet necessary change from the first book but it in no way indicates any form of "macro hierarchy". It is only for the sake of simplicity. Your body weight in kilos is roughly equal to the number of fat grams you should be consuming a day, so 1g per kilogram of bodyweight will do. Each gram of fat is going to be responsible for 9 calories of your total caloric intake.

body weight in kilograms = grams of fat per day

grams of fat per day x 9 (cals/gram) = daily calories from fat

Carbs are calculated last because they are the trickiest to calculate, not, and most people's initial estimates are too low. By forcing you to determine protein and fat first, you are left with x amount of calories to be met with carbs. (Don't worry, this calculation isn't set in stone, we will optimize and adjust in a few paragraphs). Each gram of carbohydrate is going to be responsible for 4 calories of your total caloric intake. This is where you have to do a bit more math than has been previously required.

total daily calories -(calories from fat + calories from protein) = calories from carbs

calories from carbs ÷ 4(cals/gram) = grams of carbs per day

Now you have the three numbers that comprise your daily macro profile. There is no need to count calories. Understand that by hitting these numbers, you are hitting your calories.

What Now?

Now I want you to look at the numbers you came up with and be honest with yourself and ask yourself if consistency is possible. A few things may get in the way of consistency, and the main culprit is usually your palate's preference. If you absolutely prefer carbs over fat (or vice versa) you can make the appropriate changes as long as your calories are still adding up. Try to refrain from too marked a tweak (a *tweak*, and a minor one at that, is exactly what it should be), as there is a rationale behind these initial calculations.

Exceptions To The Calculations

Protein. The common protein suggestion of "1g per pound of body weight" seems to be excessive for the majority, and should be considered as a maximum number instead. The exception being someone who is trying to gain weight, in which case it is advisable to aim for 1g per pound of *goal weight* (e.g. a 180-pound male with a goal weight of 200-pounds would aim for 200g of protein daily).

Carbs. Diabetes, PCOS, and many other diseases require a lower carb diet, in which case you should speak with a dietitian who can assist you in determining a safe and healthy carb consumption. If you suffer from a disease or illness that requires you to closely monitor carbs, a higher fat diet is absolutely acceptable.

Fat. People with digestive issues are often sensitive to fat. This can sometimes be treated by paying close attention to nutrient timing and spreading fat consumption out throughout the day. However, if you are intolerant, it is acceptable to eat a higher carb diet.

Fat Loss: Activity Level and Optimal Macro Profile

If you are attempting to lose a considerable amount of weight and your multiplier is on the lower end of the scale, it might be prudent to raise fat and lower carbs. As mentioned in Chapter Four, fat is the favored macronutrient when it comes to weight loss because it's a slower digesting nutrient whereas carbohydrates are known for being fast digesting. When eating at a deficit, you want to do everything you can to avoid hunger. If you're training less than 10 hours a week, you do not need a ton of carbohydrates.

If you sit a bit high on the multiplier scale, I do not recommend lowering your carbohydrate intake in exchange for a higher fat intake. Your body *needs* carbohydrates in order to: maintain adequate blood glucose levels, keep your CNS firing away, replenish muscle glycogen levels to fuel performance, and maintain lean body mass. If you train hard, you need carbs. Cutting them won't expedite the weight loss process because you won't be cutting calories, per se.

Which brings me to the ***caloric constraint hypothesis***. I will give a brief rundown, but I highly suggest purchasing The Renaissance Diet by Nick Shaw and Dr. Mike Israetel:

"The caloric constraint hypothesis begins with a straightforward

premise; that for any particular goal, there is a certain corresponding optimal daily calorie intake. Because calorie intake is a set value for any given goal, calorie allotment constrains the amount of all 3 of the macronutrients. This is another way of saying that if you eat more of any one of the nutrients (say protein, for example), you must necessarily eat less of one or both of the others (carbs and/or fats) to retain the optimal caloric intake.

Thus, the caloric constraint hypothesis is the statement that increasing or decreasing any particular macronutrient must come at the expense of changing one or both other macronutrients. Why is this realization important? Because it creates a framework to guide our selection of macronutrient amounts and ratios. Because the caloric constraint hypothesis (CCH) does not allow for the stand-alone raising and lowering of macronutrients."

Any shift that you make in one macro needs to be accounted for by lowering or raising the other two, whether you are cutting or maintaining (bulking is less strict, however). This is a great segue into what to do if you need to lower calories in order to accelerate weight loss, either because you calculated your deficit too low or in the event you plateau. You do not have to recalculate your macros every time you lower calories, just fat and carbs. You can lower one or the other by roughly 100g (25g carbs = 100 calories, 11g fat = 99 calories) or you can do the math and lower both by a little.

By no means should you lower your calories or macros if you didn't adhere to them consistently for 2-3 weeks. How on earth would you know your initial macro estimates weren't working if you weren't consistent?

Consistency Is The Key

The only way to truly get to know your body, is to be consistent with different approaches until you find one that works. Some people get it on the first try with their starting calculations, while some have to fuss with and tweak their macros for weeks until they have that "AH HA!" moment. I want to focus on the word consistency briefly before moving on because you are surely wondering how consistent you must be.

The most common question people seem to have upon looking at their accurately calculated daily calories and macronutrient targets is: *"How close to these numbers do I need to get?"* And my answer is the same answer I give to every training and fitness related question: *it depends*. It depends on your goal. You already know that a caloric surplus doesn't demand the same strictness as a deficit. That being said, you need to get pretty damn close to your macro numbers if you want to lose weight, but remember, flexible dieting isn't about perfection. To quote Vince Lombardi, "Perfection isn't attainable, but if we chase perfection we can catch excellence".

If you aren't getting on a stage to compete in bodybuilding any time soon, and you just want to lose a few pounds and lift some weights, don't worry too much about extreme precision. Consistency on it's own will take you far.

Getting Started

This a learning process and getting started can be the most intimidating part if you are new. Some of you may be looking at your numbers, thinking "how the fuck am I supposed to hit these dead on?" Well, since this whole thing is pretty flexible, you don't need to stress yourself out with being exact. Let's discuss how to get started in each caloric state.

Deficit. When eating at a deficit, only worry about hitting calories and protein at first, with minimal effort attempting to hit calculated carbs and fat. If you create an initial natural approach to flexible dieting, you will be able to see what you can reasonably hit every day without forcing yourself to hit your specific calculated numbers. If you can intuitively and consistently hit a different set of numbers (than initially calculated) on a daily basis and you are making progress whilst doing so, I suggest continue on with those numbers. Minor day-to-day fluctuations in carbs and fat won't hinder weight loss at all if calories are being met and a deficit is still in place. Example:

	Calories	Protein	Carbs	Fat
Calculated Numbers	1802	140	153	70
Intuitive and Consistent Numbers	1806	141	162	66

If you have extreme OCD and insist on hitting the numbers you originally calculated, you can begin to slowly dial those numbers in each day by tweaking portion sizes and food choices.

Maintenance/Athletes. When eating at maintenance, accuracy will be more beneficial for athletes since carbs and protein are crucial for performance and recovery. While protein and carb numbers should be met as closely as possible, there is more leniency for fat, and overall calories. Someone on a maintenance plan is safe fluctuating +/- 100 kcal a day given that by the end of the week, everything will end up being fairly balanced. These daily fluctuations will often come from variable fat consumption. Example:

	Calories	Protein	Carbs	Fat
Calculated Numbers	2310	170	218	84
Example One	2208	168	222	72
Example Two	2401	171	220	93

Example One: If you get to the end of your day, you've met your protein/carbs, and don't care to eat 10 grams of pure fat, don't.

Example Two: If you get to the end of the day and find that you are well below your protein goal, and a piece of steak will meet your protein allotment but put you over on fat, go for it.

These two fluctuation examples, in spite of having a difference of 21g of fat and 193 kcal between them, still fall within an acceptable +/- 100 kcal deviation from the originally calculated numbers. How's that for flexible?

Surplus. When eating at a surplus, just get the damn calories in no matter what. All that really matters is that the diet is hypercaloric and 10g fluctuations in either direction of all three macronutrients are acceptable.

	Calories	Protein	Carbs	Fat
Calculated Numbers	2900	195	314	96
Example One	2962	186	305	111
Example Two	3016	204	309	107

Despite all the fluctuations in each macro, the calories were met and the numbers were in the ballpark of the original calculation. Great success!

If flexible dieting and tracking macros is new to you, you likely won't hit each macro within a gram or two during your first few weeks of logging and tracking. Don't beat yourself up about it, just use each day as an experiment and a learning tool. You can be very relaxed or you can tighten it up. You are making the rules.

Once you get used to the tracking and logging process, there is one final step to optimize your numbers, which is to create a reasonable approach to hit your daily macronutrient needs by deciding how many meals a day best suits your lifestyle, your hunger schedule, and your preferences. This is easily done by planning ahead and having some basic knowledge of nutrient timing, and determining if it will be a useful tool or not. Strategies for effective meal planning, and a primer on nutrient timing will be covered in the following two chapters.

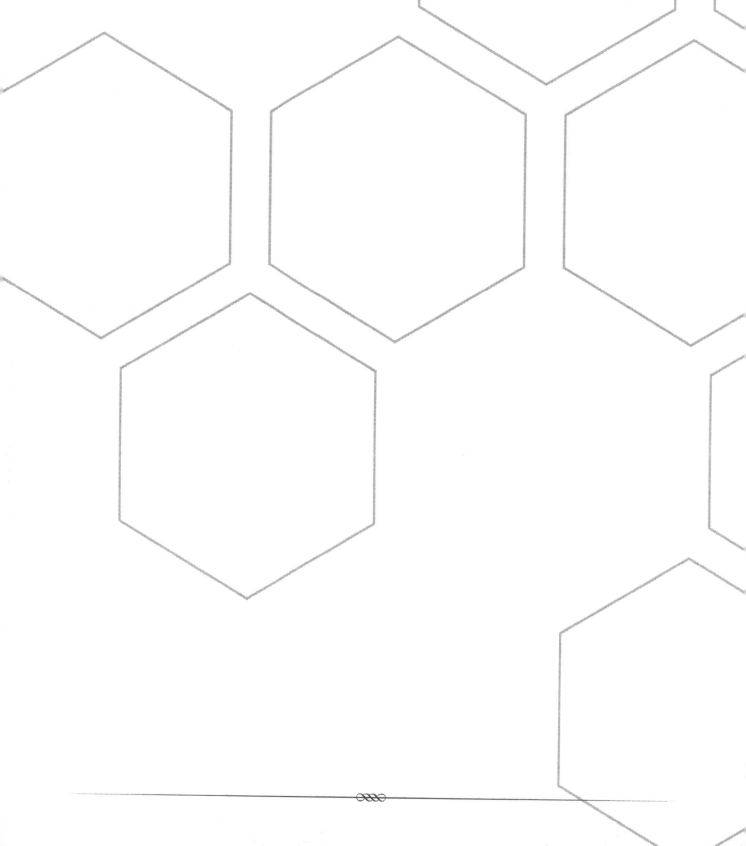

Sources & Further Reading Suggestions

Slater G, Phillips SM, authors. Nutrition guidelines for strength sports: sprinting, weightlifting, throwing events, and bodybuilding. J Sports Sci. 2011;29 Suppl 1:S67-77. doi: 10.1080/02640414.2011.574722. Epub 2011 Jun 12. Accessed at:
http://www.ncbi.nlm.nih.gov/pubmed/21660839

American Dietetic Association; Dietitians of Canada; American College of Sports Medicine, Rodriguez NR, Di Marco NM, Langley S., authors. American College of Sports Medicine position stand. Nutrition and athletic performance. Med Sci Sports Exerc. 2009 Mar;41(3):709-31. doi: 10.1249/MSS.0b013e31890eb86.
Accessed at:
http://www.ncbi.nlm.nih.gov/pubmed/19225360

Burke LM, Cox GR, Culmmings NK, Desbrow B., authors. Guidelines for daily carbohydrate intake: do athletes achieve them? Sports Med. 2001;31(4):267-99. Accessed at:
http://www.ncbi.nlm.nih.gov/pubmed/11310548

Rolls BJ, Fedoroff IC, Guthrie JF, Laster LJ, authors. Foods with different satiating effects in humans. Appetite. 1990 Oct;15(2):115-26. Accessed at:
http://www.ncbi.nlm.nih.gov/pubmed/2268137

Kissileff HR, Gruss LP, Thornton J, Jordan HA, authors. The satiating efficiency of foods. Physiol Behav. 1984 Feb;32(2):319-32. Accessed at:
http://www.ncbi.nlm.nih.gov/pubmed/6718557

Drewnowski A, authors. Energy density, palatability, and satiety: implications for weight control. Nutr Rev. 1998 Dec;56(12):347-53. Accessed at:
http://www.ncbi.nlm.nih.gov/pubmed/9884582

Phillips SM, Moore DR, Tang JE, authors. A critical examination of dietary protein requirements, benefits, and excesses in athletes. Int J Sport Nutr Exerc Metab. 2007 Aug;17 Suppl:S58-76. Accessed at:
http://www.ncbi.nlm.nih.gov/pubmed/18577776

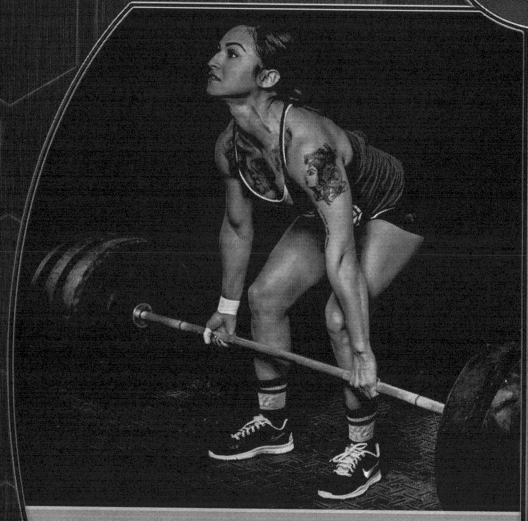

RICKLYNN LONG
CROSSFIT/ OLYMPIC WEIGHTLIFTING

RICKLYNN "LIL RIKI" LONG

WHO ARE YOU AND WHAT DO YOU DO?

MY NAME IS RICKLYNN JOY LONG, BUT EVERYONE KNOWS ME AS RIKI. I AM A DOUGHNUTS AND DEADLIFT SPONSORED ATHLETE AND I COMPETE IN OLYMPIC WEIGHTLIFTING AND CROSSFIT. WHEN I'M NOT SLANGGING WEIGHTS AND GETTING GYMNASTY, I AM COACHING ONLINE AND DROPPING KNOWLEDGE ABOUT FLEXIBLE DIETING; I AM A CERTIFIED FITNESS NUTRITION SPECIALIST.

WHEN DID YOU START FLEXIBLE DIETING AND WHY?

I FIRST DISCOVERED FLEXIBLE DIETING IN MARCH OF 2014. I HAD TRIED EVERY TYPE OF DIET POPULAR WITH CROSSFIT, BUT I ALWAYS FOUND MYSELF BINGING AND FOOD SHAMING CONSTANTLY. ONE DAY I WAS LOOKING AT PICTURES ON INSTAGRAM WITH THE HASHTAG " CLEANEATING" AND BEFORE I KNEW IT I WAS LOOKING AT A PICTURE OF A DOUGHNUT THAT HAD A HASHTAG "THEKMAEWAY." I CLICKED ON THAT HASHTAG AND FOUND KRISSY MAE CAGNEY. A WEEK LATER, SHE WAS MY FLEXIBLE DIETING COACH.

WHAT WAS YOUR DIET LIKE BEFORE FLEXIBLE DIETING?

BEFORE FLEXIBLE DIETING I WAS ATTEMPTING TO DO ANOTHER ROUND OF THE WHOLE 30 CHALLENGE, WHICH IS THE PALEO DIET BUT WITH MORE RESTRICTIONS. BEFORE THAT I DID A 21 DAY SUGAR DETOX, WHERE I WAS PROBABLY EATING HALF A POUND OF BACON, A PACK OF JERKY, SWEET POTATOES AND HALF A JAR OF ALMOND BUTTER EVERYDAY. THOUGH I WAS GETTING VERY LEAN WITH THE SUGAR DETOX, THERE WAS ABSOLUTELY NO WAY THAT I COULD EVER SUSTAIN THAT LIFESTYLE. BEFORE FLEXIBLE DIETING, IT WAS SAFE TO SAY I WAS CONVINCED THAT CARBS WERE THE ENEMY. I WAS AFRAID OF CARBS AND THOUGHT A HIGH FAT DIET WAS IDEAL.

WHAT HAS BEEN YOUR BIGGEST BREAKTHROUGH SINCE FLEXIBLE DIETING?

SINCE FLEXIBLE DIETING, THE BIGGEST BREAKTHROUGH FOR ME IS ALL THE KNOWLEDGE I HAVE GAINED ABOUT FOOD. I NOW KNOW HOW FOODS MAKE THE BODY WORK AND BECAUSE OF THAT, I NO LONGER HAVE FEAR WHEN I EAT. NO MORE FOOD SHAMING OR GUILT.

HAVE YOU USED FLEXIBLE DIETING TO PREPARE FOR A COMPETITION OR MEET?

IN A FIVE MONTH TIME FRAME, I HAD SAFELY CUT TWO WEIGHT CLASSES TO COMPETE AT THE AMERICAN OPEN AS A 48KG LIFTER. I LOST 20 POUNDS ALL THANKS TO FLEXIBLE DIETING. AS I GOT LEANER, MY STRENGTH STAYED THE SAME BECAUSE I WAS PROPERLY FUELING MY BODY WITH MY PERSONAL BALANCED MACROS. I ACTUALLY STARTED GETTING STRONGER. IN THE BEGINNING OF MY CUT AT 124 POUNDS, MY MAX SNATCH WAS 135 POUNDS; AT 105 POUND BODY WEIGHT I CAN NOW SNATCH 150 POUNDS. THERE WERE TIMES WHEN MY STRENGTH FELT TO BE DRIFTING, THAT'S WHEN I KNEW IT WAS TIME FOR A REFEEED. WITH A CONTROLLED AND STRUCTURED REFEED ABOUT EVERY TWO TO THREE WEEKS, NOT ONLY WAS I ABLE TO STAY STRONG PHYSICALLY, BUT MY MENTAL GAME WAS NEVER COMPROMISED.

WHAT ARE YOUR THREE MOST IMPORTANT GUIDELINES YOU GIVE YOURSELF WITH FLEXIBLE DIETING?

MY THREE MOST IMPORTANT GUIDELINES FOR MYSELF:
1. PLAN MY FOODS THE NIGHT BEFORE
2. IF YOU'RE REALLY HUNGRY TODAY, GO FOR VOLUME
3. PLAN YOUR BED TIME SNACK FIRST

WHAT'S THE BEST PIECE OF ADVICE FOR NEWBIES YOU WISH YOU HAD WHEN STARTING FLEXIBLE DIETING?

WELL, LUCKY FOR ME I HAD KRISSY AS MY COACH AND SHE ANSWERED EVERY SILLY QUESTIONED I HAD IN THE BEGINNING. THE ADVICE I WOULD GIVE TO THE NEWBIES THOUGH, IS TO REALLY TRUST THE PROCESS AND STICK WITH THE NUMBERS YOUR COACH GIVES YOU. IF YOU ARE CONSISTENT WITH YOUR MACROS, YOU WILL MAKE PROGRESS.

DEFINE FLEXIBLE DIETING:

I LIKE TO CALL FLEXIBLE DIETING "FLEXIBLE EATING" BECAUSE IT'S NOT EXACTLY A DIET, BUT SIMPLY MONITORING YOUR PORTIONS. THIS IS A WAY OF EATING THAT WE CAN SUSTAIN FOR THE REST OF OUR LIVES. YOU ARE GIVEN A SET OF CALORIES/MACRONUTRIENTS THAT YOU NEED TO REACH EACH DAY, AND IT IS UP TO YOU HOW YOU WANT TO HIT THOSE MACROS. WITH FLEXIBLE DIETING THERE IS NO FOOD SHAMING, NO BINGING, NO GUILT, AND OF COURSE NO RESTRICTIONS, JUST MODERATION. WITHOUT ANY RESTRICTIONS, WE ARE LESS LIKELY TO HAVE A BINGE DAY, MAKING FLEXIBLE DIETING THE BETTER CHOICE IN DIETING, PHYSICALLY, MENTALLY, AND EMOTIONALLY.

10. Tracking, Weighing & Logging Food

At this point you have your numbers calculated, and I've discussed how to slowly dial these numbers in, as well as how minor tweaking will take place in the initial phase of flexible dieting. Now you need to know how to keep track of all of this information in order to effectively put it into action.

The biggest pitfall for beginner flexible dieters is the attendant anxiety of weighing and logging food. In fact, there are many people who suggest that weighing food and tracking macros is an eating disorder in and of itself. I partially agree. Anyone who is counting almonds, attempting to track how much marinade got left in the chicken bowl, or is having a mental breakdown for being 2g over on fat would do well to remember the most important word surrounding all of this: **flexible**. Being flexible isn't being able to slam one doughnut a day in between meals consisting of lean meats and green vegetables. Being flexible is allowing the rigid rules of "weigh, track, and log everything" to bend before they break you.

If you are new to weighing food, you will need to regularly use a food scale at first, but after you weigh 6 ounces of chicken for the umpteenth time, you'll know exactly what it looks like, at which point you can omit the weighing component and just track it in your smartphone.

Which brings us to MyFitnessPal. I don't bother mentioning any other fitness-related apps, because none can come close to matching MyFitnessPal's extensive food database. There are a few other apps that are decent and designed to track macros specifically, but their food libraries are woefully inadequate compared to MFP.

The new versions of MyFitnessPal allow you to enter your exact macros, which makes tracking easier than ever. Ignore the defaults MFP tries to give you and enter what you calculate. When using MFP, it is also important to note that it is not necessary to track your activity- your activity level is already a part of your macro calculations.

Now you have your numbers registered in MFP and the tracking becomes easy thanks to the nifty barcode scanner feature. Anything you put into your mouth can be quickly recorded in your phone. You can easily see how many grams of each macro you have left for the day by simply turning your phone horizontal while navigating the "Diary" page.

The other great thing about MFP is that you can look at your entire week (rather than just one day) by going to the "Nutrition" page and selecting "Weekly". This is an excellent way to see if the minor macro-fluctuations that occur on a daily basis balance out over the course of a week, which is the ultimate goal when it comes to measuring consistency.

The app makes the logging and tracking process very easy on the user. All that's required from the user is consistency and accuracy.

CONSISTENCY. At first, you should be tracking daily, and tracking everything as accurately as possible. If you are tracking daily, you are being held accountable to see what you are eating since the app gives you a visual. This is usually an eye opener as this is when you may see just how much you were previously over or under eating. Consistently tracking will prevent you from continuing to over or under eat. This is also going to teach you to look at food labels, understand the make-up of different foods, and keep your macronutrients in check.

ACCURACY. You need to enter the correct portion size for the app to accurately track it. Every food has a "serving suggestion" or a "standard serving size", which can be used in place of an exact measurement, or, if you have an exact measurement, enter it directly into the app, which will do the math for you. If you eat 7 ounces of salmon, but fail to change the 3.5 ounce serving suggestion in the app, you'll end up with an inaccurate inventory of calories, protein, and fat for the day. Weighing and measuring food is a pain in the ass, but the best way to become a pro at "eyeballing" food is by weighing and measuring it. Just like with everything else, practice makes perfect. If you are coming off of a "clean" or "bro" diet, you are probably fairly good at weighing and measuring (at least something good came from it). Again, your measurements do not need to be exact, but you need to make an honest and concerted effort.

Planning Ahead

Nobody wants to be "that guy" who is frantically scanning food into a smartphone in public, then spending 10 minutes doing math afterward. Having a plan is always suggested. Most people plan their training out a week (usually more) in advanced, so why not plan your nutrition?

Many of you may own my meal prep book, *This Is Not A Cookbook*. In the book I stress the importance of planning ahead, and how to do it. Whether you meal prep or food prep (the differences are explained in the book) for the following day or the next six days, having a plan is a tremendous aid to staying on track.

It takes a lot of practice and experience with macros to be able to "wing it", day in and day out, successfully. I have been doing this a long time and I still like to plan at least a day ahead in order to hit my goals. You may be the type of person who needs to plan their entire week out, or you may be the type to figure it out the night before. Either way, I strongly advise that you plan ahead in order to make this a little easier on yourself in the early stages. On the days where you end up winging it, you'll notice that you are often left with a ton of carbs or protein at the end of each day. When this happens, you feel like you're stuck eating fruit (sugar) to fill your carbs, or egg whites to fill your protein. This is neither fun, nor conducive to reaching your goals.

Try entering your food the night before. Take your schedule into consideration and enter the food you know you will be consuming, for instance: leftovers in the fridge, pre/post workout meals, and what you have available to cook, then make a plan. This is a surefire way to hit your macros without screwing yourself come night time by blindly tracking over the course of the day. Added bonus: doing this will likely save you money. There is a weird phenomenon that I like to call "*I Already Tracked It So I Have To Fucking Eat It*" that occurs when you practice tracking ahead that prevents you from spending money eating out, or making pointless trips to the grocery store where you end up spending $72 on a snack run for gummy bears, cookie dough, hummus, and Vaseline. I don't know what the hell you need the Vaseline for, but who am I to judge.

Upon getting your most important meals entered, you are left with some wiggle room and can still be flexible (but not so flexible that you get off track). Seeing your whole day ahead of time gives you the upper hand.

Pre-entering also familiarizes you even more with portion sizes. You'll start to know exactly what 5 ounces of ground beef, 3 ounces of sweet potato, and 2 tablespoons of peanut butter all look like and how each fills up your macros. Being able to visually measure your portions will benefit you immensely at times when you may not actually be able to measure, eating out for example.

Now that you have an overall understanding of how to calculate, tweak, and track all your numbers (all while remaining flexible) we are going to focus on the details.

A Step-by-Step Guide to Planning Your Meals One Week at a Time

1. Download MyFitnessPal on to your phone and change your daily macros to the ones you have been given. You will get far more out of this app if you purchase the premium package for $50. This one time purchase is more than worth it as you can enter exact macros by the gram and have multiple sets of macros in order to track properly on training days, rest days, etc. If you opt not to go premium, you will have one set of macros that is based off a percentage opposed to exact grams and you will need to be OK with remembering rest day and training day macros. If you are unfamiliar with the ins and outs of MFP, watch the provided tutorial and play around with the app by scanning items in and using some of the features.

2. The most important thing to consider when planning your nutrition is determining a practical and realistic approach. The "wing it" approach is extremely inconsistent and can be stressful, as you'll spend more time doing math and playing macro Tetris than you spend in the gym. Set 20-30 minutes aside on Sunday to get ready for the week ahead.

3. The first step is determining how many core meals (meaning full meals, not snacks) you want to eat a day; there is no right or wrong answer here. Some people do better on two large meals a day and others do better on four. The important thing is to choose the route that will keep you both happy and consistent. You can name your meals in MFP; I highly suggest you do that.

4. Looking at your macros and number of desired core meals, start planning your meals ahead for the week. Enter what you KNOW you will eat each day. Save common meals on MFP to make this easier, this way you won't need to manually enter each day. You can copy any meal to any day. Create and save meals on Sunday night, then you can easily add them throughout the week. Know that you can tweak and adjust meals; the serving sizes aren't set in stone. For example if you save a meal in your phone that has 5 ounces of chicken in it, once you add it to a day in your food diary, you can easily change that serving size to 6 ounces if need be.

5. Create a training day menu and a rest day menu. On training days you will have pre and post workout meals containing carbs. Beyond that, consider your training time. If you training in the morning, you should consider incorporating more carbs into breakfast. If you training in the evening, you should consider incorporating more carbs into dinner. On rest days, your carb intake will be lower and fat intake will be higher. Rest days typically mean fattier cuts of meat/fish, which is something to take into account when planning for the week. Here are some basics to keep in mind:
   - Protein: Should be broken up evenly based on your meal schedule & consumed through the day.
   - Fat: Slowest digesting macro and keeps you satisfied the longest. Consume a bulk of your fat when you tend to get the hungriest during the day.
   - Carbs: Human gasoline. Seventy percent should be consumed around your training time. For example, "bookend" your training with roughly 35% before and 35% after. Do not overthink this guideline.
   - Fiber: Roughly 15% of your daily carbohydrate intake should come from fiber. By consuming adequate fiber, it will be virtually impossible to over consume sugar.

6. Add any supplements that you take daily in order to be accurate with micronutrients and calories (vitamins, BCAAs, protein, etc.).

7. Give your plan a once over to make sure macros and micros are met. If your micronutrients are under 100%, go back and add more produce

8. Head to the grocery store once you have your nutrition outlined. Buy all the food you have entered for the week and then some. See provide shopping list.

9. Prep some food to make life easier. For example, making a big pot of rice at the beginning of the week will make eating a hell of a lot easier. If you want to actually prep and portion your meals to keep you on track, go for it. Make sure you buy high quality Tupperware in order for your food to keep better.

10. Set alarms on your phone during the day if you are prone to under eating or forgetting to eat (athletes are busy people). Skipping meals is completely fine because meal timing plays a very minimal role in the grand scheme of

things, however over eating at the end of the day because you forgot to eat will make most people miserable.

11.   If you know you will be going out to eat at any point in the week, look at the menu ahead of time and assess your options. Enter as much as possible ahead of time in order to make eating during the day easier. The more you have entered ahead of time, the easier nutrition will be. Remove the guesswork, remove the stress!

12.   You will almost always have "left over macros" that are unaccounted for each day after planning out your meals. This gives you options. For example, if you are hungrier than you anticipated you would be, you have some wiggle room for bigger servings. You can divvy them up between snacks throughout the day, or you can save them till the end of the day in hopes to squeeze in another meal of your liking.

13.   At the end of the day, if your calories, protein, and micros are closely met, you did well. The whole point of this is flexibility and leniency and we never want perfect to be the enemy of the good. The more you plan, track, and measure, the easier this will become for you. The planning ahead part is usually what is the most stressful part for people but after a few weeks of practice, it will start to come easy.

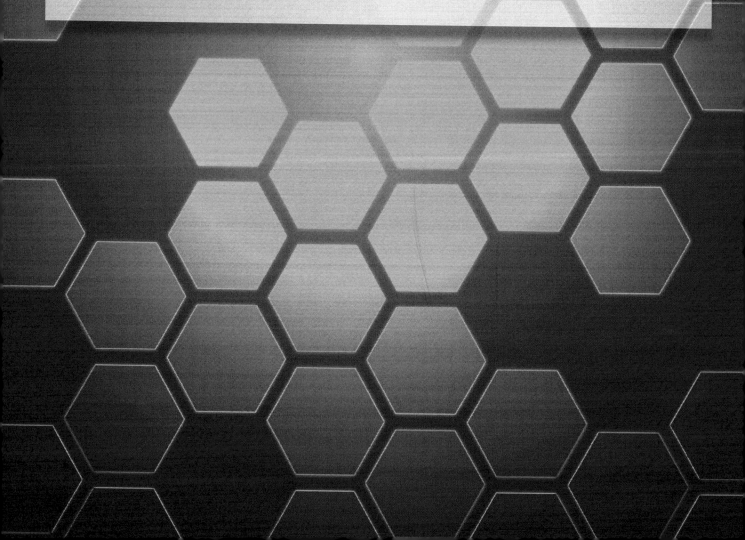

11. Nutrient Timing

Nutrient timing is easily the most controversial aspect of nutrition. In short, nutrient timing suggests that there are not only optimal times of the day to eat, but optimal times to eat specific macronutrients, as well. This nutrient schedule usually revolves around training time. An exhaustive discussion of such a complex topic would not be possible in the span of a few pages. This brief rundown will give you a good starting point, and should you find yourself keen to learn more, the suggested reading material mentioned throughout the chapter will help you in your elective research. Before we jump into who can benefit from nutrient timing (and when), I want to clear something up about meal frequency, as it usually falls into the "nutrient timing" category.

Meal Frequency

"Six small meals a day", they said, "you'll get lean", they said. You've surely heard that consuming several small meals, timed perfectly throughout the day "boosts your metabolism", or my personal favorite: "eating every two hours tricks your body into burning more calories!". The human body is a complex organism that has evolved over the course of millions of years, and is well-adapted to survive in extreme circumstances. It's metabolism is not easily "tricked", especially by high frequency meal plans. Most people do not have the time to eat every few hours throughout the day on a set schedule. In fact, these types of plans are reminiscent of the kinds of rigid meal plans that we are trying to liberate ourselves from.

Both anecdotal and clinical evidence has shown that, whether it's three meals or eight meals a day (and everything in between), meal frequency isn't the biggest determinant of long-term diet success. What does this mean for you? Choose a meal frequency that allows consistency, accuracy, and (most importantly) flexibility.

> *"Several epidemiological studies have observed an inverse relationship between people's habitual frequency of eating and body weight, leading to the suggestion that a 'nibbling' meal pattern may help in the avoidance of obesity. We conclude that the epidemiological evidence is at best very weak, and almost certainly represents an artefact. A detailed review of the possible mechanistic explanations for a metabolic advantage of nibbling meal patterns failed to reveal significant benefits in respect of energy expenditure. We conclude that any effects of meal pattern on the regulation of body weight are likely to be mediated through effects on the food intake side of the energy balance equation."*[12]

Plan on eating when you are hungry and eating until you are full. Science proves, and practicality demands that you should eat when it best suits you. So you can take the notion of small, frequent meals being optimal

---

12   Bellisle F1, McDevitt R, Prentice AM., authors. Meal frequency and energy balance [Internet]. Br J Nutr. 1997 Apr;77 Suppl 1:S57-70. Accessed at: http://www.ncbi.nlm.nih.gov/pubmed/9155494

for the physique, tie it to a rock, and toss it into a lake. Hitting your calories and macros is far more important than attempting to optimize meal timing based on planetary alignment, the Mayan calendar, and other nonsense.

I personally like to have 4 meals a day, which includes my pre and post-workout meals. I don't have a set training time each day, so sometimes breakfast serves as my pre-workout, and sometimes dinner serves as post workout. By allowing myself to be flexible with my approach, I don't need to meticulously plan to eat at a certain time each day and I am able to train whenever time allows. Even after four meals, I usually do have some leftover macros that I use to enjoy a treat at some point during the day, or a protein bar for the days I am exceptionally busy and need to stay fueled while I am on the go.

Once you decide how many meals a day is realistic, you can start thinking about the minute details of nutrient timing. Note: *you should not be worrying about nutrient timing before consistently being able to hit your calories and macros on a daily, or weekly, basis.*

> *"A deviation from optimal calorie balance can make or break a diet goal. A deviation from macronutrient amounts, especially protein intake, can seriously hinder goals. But a deviation from optimal timing will only have at most a small effect on the results of a program."* -Shaw/Israetel

Macronutrient Timing

Nutrient timing has its time and place. It typically won't accelerate results for anyone with general weight loss goals; however, athletes can benefit greatly from it, especially during competition. Nutrient timing must be planned *carefully* in order to enhance athletic performance.

NUTRIENT TIMING

THE IMPORTANCE OF NUTRIENT TIMING IS A PRIORITY-BASED CONTINUUM. THERE ARE TWO FACTORS THAT AFFECT THE PRIORITIZATION OF NUTIENT TIMING: THE SCALE OF TIME FOR THE INDIVIDUAL GOAL, AND THE INTENSITY OF EFFORT IT TAKES TO ACHEIVE THAT GOAL. FOR GENERAL WEIGHT GAIN OR LOSS, OR ANY LONGER TERM GOAL, THE PRIORITY REMAINS LOW, AND APPROACHES MODERATE PRIORITY FOR EXTREME CASES.

THE PRIORITY FOR NUTRIENT TIMING ALSO REMAINS LOW FOR NOVICE ATHLETES OR GENERAL FITNESS AND FOR NON-ENDURANCE ACTIVITIES AS WELL. FOR ENDURANCE EVENTS AND PROFESSIONALS, PRIORITY IS HIGH. HERE WE DIVIDE THIS CONTINUUM INTO LONG TERM GOALS (CHANGING WEIGHT OVER THE COURSE OF WEEKS DOWN TO DAYS) AND THE SECOND EXAMINES THE PRIORITY FOR NUTRIENT TIMING FOR SPECIFIC ATHLETIC ENDEAVORS.

NUTRIENT TIMING PRIORITY FOR BODY COMPOSITION

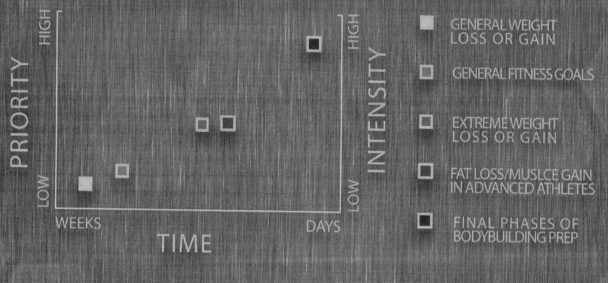

NUTRIENT TIMING PRIORITY FOR PERFORMANCE

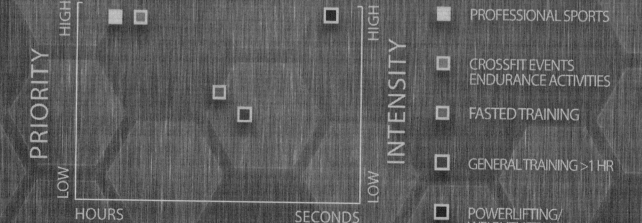

ADAPTED FROM ALAN ARAGON'S *CONTINUUM OF NUTRIENT TIMING IMPORTANCE* (WWW.ALANARAGON.COM)

*What nutrient timing **is** important for*: multiple training sessions a day, very intense long lasting exercise, physical competitions (meets, games, etc.)

*What nutrient timing is **not** important for*: general weight loss, body composition of novice lifters, general health.

Protein. Protein and amino acids are responsible for our lean body mass. Our tissues grow and shrink over days, weeks, months, and years depending on our nutrition, training, and activity levels. I think that it's safe to assume that most people have a goal of either preserving or increasing muscle tissue mass, which is why we must ingest an adequate amount of protein, but when should it be ingested?

We need protein for a variety of reasons beyond building muscle, as it is required by other cells for integrity and repair. If protein consumption is inadequate, our body will recruit amino acids from the only available source: muscle tissue. That being said, protein (or amino acids in general) is the macronutrient that should be introduced into our system regularly throughout the day in order to maximize muscle protein synthesis. The synthesis of muscle protein is vital to the body's continuing repair, development, and maintenance of its skeletal muscle groups.[13]

Long story short, do not attempt to eat all you protein at once in large amounts, rather spread it out even throughout the course of the day by evenly distributing it into your chosen approach of meal frequency. For example, if you are consuming 160g of protein a day and you have opted to have 4 meals a day, you should aim for 40g protein per meal. Whereas if you have opted to have 6 meals a day, aim for 25-30g protein per meal. Another reason to spread out protein intake is to give your organs a chance to actually digest everything you are consuming.

13   The Gale Group. Muscle Protein Synthesis.Advantmeg Inc. Accessed 5 January 2015 at: http://www.faqs.org/sports-science/Mo-Pl/Muscle-Protein-Synthesis.html

Lastly, we must discuss protein timing in regard to training and activity. If you are consuming protein regularly throughout your day, you don't need to worry too much about timing in relation to activity as you have a steady supply of amino acids coming in. One of your planned meals will usually end up being your post workout. Once muscle breakdown starts taking place from activity, introducing more protein can stop the process, but it doesn't have to come in a Blender Bottle. There is no need to consume a protein shake within 5 minutes of a workout if you aren't an advanced lifter or athlete. Keep in mind that muscle repair won't take place in the minutes following training, but in the days following. If you are attempting to lose weight and are on a large deficit, pass on drinking any calories and just eat a meal. Your meal is based completely on preference, some people enjoy elaborate protein smoothies with all the fixings and some people just want a plate of hot food.

That being said the following people may benefit from consuming intra or post workout protein supplement (the kind that comes in a Blender Bottle): those who have very long, intense training sessions, those partaking in long athletic events, or those who train fasted in the morning.

Carbs. Unlike protein, our bodies are able to store carbohydrates in our muscles and liver for later use. This means that frequency doesn't matter, but there is some interesting stuff to be said about carbohydrate timing in relation to training time. You have probably been told to consume you carbs around your training time, and there is a good reason why. As discussed in Chapter Five, your body prefers to run on glycogen.

By consuming carbs *before* you train, the following transpires:

- Muscle glycogen stores are topped off.
- Intense training recruits the CNS, which prefers carbohydrates ahead of protein or fat. Limiting carb intake may inhibit neural drive.
- When glycogen and blood glucose are present, the body will not burn muscle for fuel.

How many grams of carbs should you consume prior to training? A safe suggestion is to consume 30-40% of your daily carbs in the three hours prior to training. You can spread them out if you prefer to graze, or you can have a hefty meal and eat them in one sitting. One thing to keep in mind is that the digestive process is physiologically demanding, so if you eat too close to you training time, your body will have to find the energy to digest your food AND train. The food coma is real. In addition, it is pointless to have your meal sitting in your gut when you train as the nutrients haven't been absorbed yet, which defeats the entire purpose of the meal.

Some athletes benefit from intra-workout nutrition. I am going to plug The Renaissance Diet for the umpteenth time because that should be the next book every serious athlete reads after this one (if you haven't scooped it up already). Nick and Mike wrote pages about intra-workout carb consumptions, but that is not the focus of this book, hence why I am directing you there. There is an extensive chapter on nutrient timing for athletes that expands upon a lot of what I am briefly trying to cover here.

Lastly, we have post-workout carb consumption, which is just as important as pre-workout consumption if you are a serious athlete. The evidence supporting the benefit of post-workout carbs is overwhelming. The benefits include, but are not limited to:

- Glycogen replenishment[14]
- Anti-catabolism
- Insulin spiking (insulin is an anabolic hormone for human tissue)

I suggest that my athletes consume about 40% of their daily carbohydrates after training (the two hours immediately following training). If you are consuming a large quantity of carbs on a daily basis, that may be a

---

14   Gregory Tardie, Ph.D. author. Glycogen Replenishment After Exhaustive Exercise. United States Sports Academy. 2008 Feb 11. Accessed from The Sports Journal at: http://thesportjournal. org/article/glycogen-replenishment-after-exhaustive-exercise/

lot to get down in one sitting, in which case you can drink half of them and eat the other half once you are able to eat a meal.

There is a reason why carbs have a bad reputation. Once you consume too many carbs in one sitting (or over the course of a day) and your glycogen stores are full, the excess gets stored in the form of fat. If you are consuming 30-40% of your carbs prior to training and 40% after training, that leaves you with 20-30% to spread out during the rest of your day, which isn't going to pack any pounds on your physique (unless that's your goal, and your carb calculations demonstrate this fact well).

Fat. Fat, like carbs, can be stored in our bodies for later use, but in the form of adipose tissue. The good news is that fat timing is relatively simple in comparison to carb and protein timing.

As we already know, fat is extremely slow digesting, which means the only time it should really be avoided is prior to training (or at least make sure you give it enough time to digest). The only "rule" I suggest is to eat a high fat meal at the point in your day when you tend to be hungriest, or when you know you will have to go a long period of time without a meal.

One Scenario Worth Mentioning

There is one type of person who tends to have some trouble with nutrient timing, and that is the crazy person who has the motivation to wake up at 4am and train. The early risers tend to have a tough time with pre-workout meals because they usually train this early out of necessity, rather than desire, which means a time crunch is present. If you are a morning person, try to shove a banana down your throat (uh, phrasing?) en route to the gym. If food is out of the question before an early morning training session, you should instead try to have your last meal of each day right before bed, making sure it has enough fat to slow down digestion of carbs and protein. This will prime you for your ass-crack-of-dawn training sessions.

Keep in mind that everything mentioned above is a loose guideline, and you by no means should be stressing yourself out about the perfect way to apportion out your daily allotments of protein, carbs, and fat. When you start focussing on nutrient timing too much, you lose sight of being flexible. The people who benefit from nutrient timing are primarily performance athletes (and nutrition nerds).

I mentioned previously that I try to have four meals a day, and I have a simple approach when it comes to apportioning my macros across those meals. I try to "bookend" my training with meals consisting of protein/carbs and the two meals farthest away from my training are protein/fat dominant. Example:

	Meal One	Meal Two	Meal Three	Meal Four
AM Training	Protein/Carbs	Protein/Carbs	Protein/Fat	Protein/Fat
Noon Training	Protein/Fat	Protein/Carbs	Protein/Carbs	Protein/Fat
PM Training	Protein/Fat	Protein/Fat	Protein/Carbs	Protein/Carbs

Of course my meals will have trace amounts of the macros not mentioned, but I make an effort to get the bulk of my carbs into the two meals on each end of my training. One more thing I want to add, is that this schedule isn't taking snacks into account. My "leftover" macros get spent on treats or snacks which I just eat when I am hungry. This is what flexible means to me.

Numbers will **always** have the largest impact on the physiological components that alter body composition (however, you can get away with more as a performance athlete). This is why "If It Fits Your Macros" works for getting lean. However, if you are someone who takes their diet and training seriously, you already know that intelligent food choices must take precedent in order to aid the systems of your body and general overall health.

Sources & Further Reading Suggestions:

Brad Jon Schoenfeld1, Alan Albert Aragon and James W Krieger, authors. The effect of protein timing on muscle strength and hypertrophy: a meta-analysis. Journal of the International Society of Sports Nutrition 2013, 10:53 doi:10.1186/1550-2783-10-53. Accessed at:
http://www.jissn.com/content/10/1/53

Lemon PW1, Berardi JM, Noreen EE., authors. The role of protein and amino acid supplements in the athlete's diet: does type or timing of ingestion matter? Curr Sports Med Rep. 2002 Aug;1(4):214-21. Accessed at:
http://www.ncbi.nlm.nih.gov/pubmed/12831698

Chad Kerksick, Travis Harvey, Jeff Stout, Bill Campbell, Colin Wilborn, Richard Kreider, Doug Kalman, Tim Ziegenfuss, Hector Lopez, Jamie Landis, John L Ivy and Jose Antonio, authors. International Society of Sports Nutrition position stand: Nutrienttiming. Journal of the International Societyof Sports Nutrition. 2008 October 3. Accessed at:
http://www.biomedcentral.com/content/pdf/1550-2783-5-17.pdfJournal

Blake B. Rasmussen , Kevin D. Tipton , Sharon L. Miller , Steven E. Wolf , Robert R. Wolfe, authors. An oral essential amino acid-carbohydrate supplement enhances muscle protein anabolism after resistance exercise.Journal of Applied Physiology Published 1 February 2000 Vol. 88 no. 2, 386-392. Accessed at:
http://jap.physiology.org/content/88/2/386

Alan Albert Aragon and Brad Jon Schoenfeld, authors. Nutrient timing revisited: is there a post-exercise anabolic window? Journal of the International Society of Sports Nutrition 2013, 10:5 doi:10.1186/1550-2783-10-5 Published: 29 January 2013. Accessed at: http://www.jissn.com/content/10/1/5

S. M. Phillips , K. D. Tipton , A. Aarsland , S. E. Wolf , R. R. Wolfe, authors. Mixed muscle protein synthesis and breakdown after resistance exercise in humans.
American Journal of Physiology - Endocrinology and Metabolism Published 1 July 1997 Vol. 273 no. 1, E99-E107. Accessed at:
http://ajpendo.physiology.org/content/273/1/E99.short

Dr. Layne Norton, author. Optimal protein intake to maximize muscle protein synthesis: Examinations of optimal meal protein intake and frequency for athletes. AgroFOOD Industry Hi-Tech 2009 March/April. pp. 54-57. Accessed at:
http://www.biolayne.com/wp-content/uploads/Norton-J-Ag-Food-Ind-Hi-Tech-2008.pdf

Kerksick C1, Harvey T, Stout J, Campbell B, Wilborn C, Kreider R, Kalman D, Ziegenfuss T, Lopez H, Landis J, Ivy JL, Antonio J, authors. International Society of Sports Nutrition position stand: nutrient timing. J Int Soc Sports Nutr. 2008 Oct 3;5:17. doi: 10.1186/1550-2783-5-17. Accessed at:
http://www.ncbi.nlm.nih.gov/pubmed/1883450

12. Food Selection & Composition

From an aesthetic standpoint, food composition plays little to no role in your body composition (this is why people can get lean eating non-nutrient dense, calorically dense food). If your goals are primarily health and/or performance related, you should be consuming nutrient dense, high quality foods a majority of the time. Treat your body well. There is plenty of room for doughnuts and ice cream occasionally, but a bulk of your food should definitely come from high quality proteins, healthy fats, vegetables, and other things that come from the earth, and not a factory. Eat a lot of whole, minimally processed, filling foods that are rich in vitamins and minerals. Eat the "fun" stuff when you want to if you have the caloric room for it.

If you are logging into MFP and your vitamins, calcium, and iron are not at 100% that is a good indicator that you are eating like an asshole and you should start making some better choices.

"It's generally better to focus on improving your food quality before your food quantity, as this often helps you control your

MACRO BREAKDOWNS

REFLECTS BOTH THE CALORIC LOAD AS WELL AS THE MACRO BREAKDOWNS OF A FEW FOODS. NOTE: GROUND BEEF IS 80% LEAN 20% FAT BY WEIGHT, NOT BY CALORIES

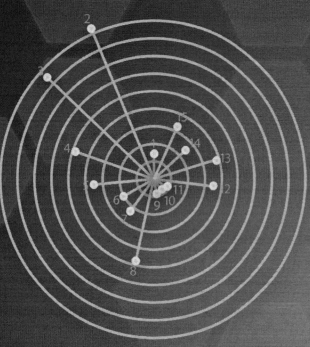

1. EGG: 71 cal
2. RIBEYE (6 oz): 462 cals
3. 80/20 GROUND BEEF (6 oz): 426 cals
4. SALMON (6 oz): 242 cals
5. SKINLESS CHICKEN BREAST (6 oz): 186 cals
6. 0% GREEK YOGURT (6 oz): 100 cals
7. BANANA (7-8"): 105 cals
8. WHITE RICE (½ cup uncooked): 242 cals
9. KALE (1 cup): 33 cals
10. ASPARAGUS (6 SPEARS): 24 cals
11. BELL PEPPER (1 cup): 30 cals
12. PISTACHIOS (¼ cup): 171 cals
13. PEANUT BUTTER (2 tbsp): 188 cals
14. AVOCADO (½ of fruit): 114 cals
15. OREOS (3 cookies (uh huh sure)): 160 cals

PROTEIN   FAT   CARBS

1. 35%   EGG   65%
2. 27%   RIBEYE   73%
3. 29%   80/20 GROUND BEEF   71%
4. 58%   SALMON   42%
5. 90%   SKINLESS CHICKEN BREAST   10%
6. 72%   0% GREEK YOGURT   28%
7. 7%   BANANA   93%
8. 10%   WHITE RICE   90%
9. 16%   12%   KALE   72%
10. 40%   20% ASPARAGUS   40%
11. 17%   BELL PEPPER   83%
12. 13%   67% PISTACHIOS   20%
13. 15%   72% PEANUT BUTTER   13%
14. 4%   73% AVOCADO   19%
15. 2%   38% OREOS   60%

food intake by default." -Armi Legge

It is time to learn more about the make-up of food and how to make the best choices based upon your goals and your macros. If you are on "poverty macros" you can't get away with eating too much of the fun stuff. Unless your diet consists entirely of lean meat and green vegetables, you won't be poppin' stacks of Oreos on a day-to-day basis. On the contrary, if you are on "hood rich macros" (aka "yolo macros" aka "Dan Bilzerian macros") you can get away with eating just about anything you damn well please. The chances are you would get sick if you tried to cram 4000 kcal of chicken and vegetables down your gob.

Tips For Food Choices On A Deficit

If you're on a deficit, avoid drinking your calories at all costs. Start by tightening up your coffee fixings followed by eliminating protein shakes if need be. Drinking your calories will not accelerate fat loss and it can also leave you hungry by the end of the day. Protein shakes work well when you are chronically deficient in protein for whatever reason, but beyond that, they are not at all necessary when cutting weight. If you drink a 200 calorie shake that will be digested in under an hour, you are doing yourself a great disservice as those are precious calories that could have been savored, chewed, and would have kept you satisfied longer.

You should aim to fill your diet up with non-calorically dense foods that are high volume and highly satiating. Any foods with a high water content, rich micronutrient profile, high fiber content, or are "heavy" (in terms of weight) are going to be your best friend (potatoes for example, along with other root vegetables). Protein and carb selection is very important when on a cut since you want to get the biggest bang for your caloric buck. Four ounces of ribeye is going to yield substantially more calories than four ounces of chicken breast. The more intelligent your food choices, the more room for occasional indulgences when you want (or need) one. One day you may really want that ribeye instead of chicken, but one day you may want to save that fat for some peanut butter. Good thing you know how to account for both choices through flexible dieting.

Being on a cut is only as hard as you make it out to be. As discussed in previous chapters, protein and overall caloric consumption are the biggest variables to which the most attention should be paid. Beyond that use the information in this chapter to make smart decisions in order to be healthy, feel good, perform well in the gym, and not kill anyone because you are "*hangry*".

Tips For Food Choices On A Surplus

There are two types of people who are on a surplus: those who love it, and those who are wussies. The former has no problem consuming mass quantities of food and loves the process as he or she understands that this is only temporary, so they enjoy the feeding frenzy while its allowed. The latter usually tries to be overly healthy by only consuming nutrient dense foods throughout the day. There is nothing wrong with consuming a lot of nutrient dense foods . . . until you have to consume thousands of calories worth and most people don't handle that type of food volume well. Feeling uncomfortably full all day long is like an all-day commute on the struggle bus.

If you are having a difficult time consuming as many calories as you need in order to gain weight, start drinking your calories (shakes, smoothies, etc.) because they digest much faster and will give your stomach a break. Large meals consisting of grass fed beef, sweet potatoes, and a pounds of brussel sprouts can sit in your stomach for upward of 7 hours. This won't feel great when you're forced to pile more food on top.

It is alright to give yourself some leniency. Should you be consuming your 400 grams of carbs by eating a whole box of cereal followed by a bag of sour gummies? Please don't. Your mouth will hurt. But more importantly, you're not doing much for your internal health by getting high on sugar. Instead, have ¼ the box, a handful of gummies (a normal hand, not Andre the Giant-sized), a cup of quinoa, and some fiber rich produce.

There are numerous ways to approach meal design, but it all starts with knowing what food options you have available when it comes to choosing proteins, carbs, and fats. It is important to remember to look at food in its entirety as opposed to a singular respective macro. Most foods will have an overlap of macros, although one will usually be dominant.

Protein. There are many different types of protein. Different types will yield different volumes of protein, as well as vary in digestion times. Animal protein has the highest bioavailability or "biological value". Dairy is an animal byproduct and isn't necessarily considered animal protein.

> *"Biological value measures protein quality by calculating the nitrogen used for tissue formation divided by the nitrogen absorbed from food. This product is multiplied by 100 and expressed as a percentage of nitrogen utilized. The biological value provides a measurement of how efficient the body utilizes protein consumed in the diet. A food with a high value correlates to a high supply of the essential amino acids. **Animal sources typically possess a higher biological value than vegetable sources due to the vegetable source's lack of one or more of the essential amino acids.**"*[15]

• Animal protein includes beef, poultry, fish, shellfish, seafood, pork, eggs and wild game. More commonly known as "meat", animal protein tends

---

15   Jay R. Hoffman and Michael J. Falvo, authors. PROTEIN – WHICH IS BEST? [Internet archive] International Society of Sports Nutrition Symposium, June 18-19, 2005, Las Vegas NV, USA - Symposium - Macronutrient Utilization During Exercise: Implications For Performance And Supplementation. Journal of Sports Science and Medicine (2004) 3, 118-130. Accessed at: http://www.jssm.org/vol3/n3/2/v3n3-2pdf.pdf

to be fairly slow digesting.

- Dairy protein includes cheese, milk, and yogurt, and is the slowest digesting protein due to the fact that casein is present.
- Plant protein includes all protein sources that come from the agriculture such as the small amount of protein present in foods such as legumes, grains, and vegetables.
- Supplemented protein includes whey isolate, whey concentrate, casein, plant based, soy, pea, and hemp. Supplemented protein, since it comes in the form of powder, is very fast digesting.

Most protein has a fat component that you will ingest with it (aside from some supplements, egg whites, and some seafood), which will slow digestion down substantially.

Carbohydrates. Carbs are usually where you get to be the most flexible since there are a wide array carb-rich options. Carbs include food such as potatoes, yams, rice products, beans, squash, legumes, nuts, wheat products, lentils, quinoa, oats, corn, sugar, fruit, leafy greens, and vegetables.

I didn't list specifics, as there are literally hundreds of foods that can fall into the "wheat products" category (almost every processed food you can find in a grocery store), which includes foods like pastas, breads, cereals, crackers, and cookies, for example.

I also didn't give you a list of fruits and vegetables because this book isn't meant to give you a list of foods to choose from. This is meant to teach you a better way and how to explore the veritable cornucopia of options that you have available to you.

There are multiple types of carbs: starchy, sugary, and fibrous. The sugary carbs (also known as simple carbs) are fastest digesting, thus they will provide a quick burst of energy as well as replenish glycogen stores quicker than other carbs. Sugary carbs, with the exception of fruit, contain scant amounts of micronutrients, and are not suggested in excess for your overall health, however they are completely acceptable in moderation each day. Fibrous carbs are very slow digesting; when you need to stay full for a long time, fiber will do the trick. Vegetables are the best source of fiber.

It should be noted that carbohydrates and fat tend to overlap the most (for example nuts, avocado, and baked goods).

Fat. Like protein and carbs, there are several types of fat to choose from. Some dietary fat is much more beneficial from an internal health standpoint than others, and usually falls into two categories:

- Saturated fats include animal fats and coconut products (which are known as the healthier options). Beyond that, saturated fat also comes from animal byproducts like eggs, dairy, and butter.
- Unsaturated fats include the healthier monounsaturated (avocados, nuts, nut butters, olive oil) and polyunsaturated (vegetable oils).

Not mentioned are trans fats because you should stay the hell away from that processed garbage. Most people think *Partially Hydrogenated Oil* means "trans fat" but that is not necessarily the case. It is also worth noting that "healthy" oils such as canola are processed in factories, contain trans fats, and is heated to a high temperature-which can oxidize the fat and cause all sorts of health problems.

This vs. That

Here is a table with the macronutrient profiles of two mystery foods. One is an apple with a tablespoon of all natural peanut butter, and the other is an Original Glazed Doughnut® from Krispy Kreme. Can you guess which is which?

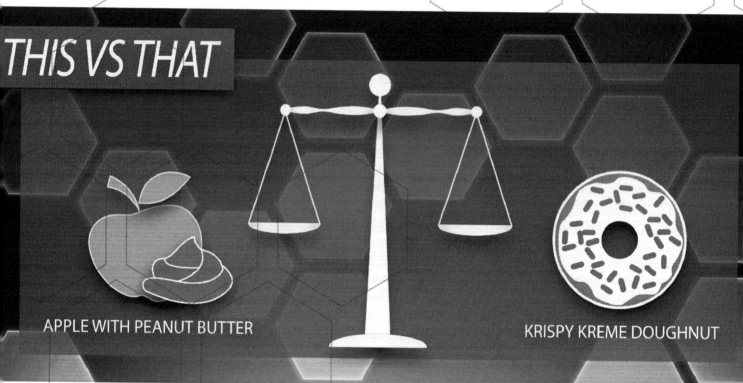

THIS VS THAT

APPLE WITH PEANUT BUTTER

KRISPY KREME DOUGHNUT

	Calories	Protein	Carbs	Fat	Sugar
Food A	241	5	35	9	25
Food B	187	2	21	11	10

Food A is the apple and peanut butter, which has 30% more calories and nearly double the sugar content of the Krispy Kreme Original Glazed Doughnut®. Before you throw the book down and start firing off hate e-mails, understand that I am in no way advocating eating a doughnut over a piece of fruit. The comparison is merely to illustrate the point that, from a caloric standpoint, you can get away with eating a doughnut every now and again if it makes you happy. Your progress won't be negatively affected, especially if that doughnut will prevent a binge that you've been on the brink of from prolonged caloric restriction; so choose the doughnut over the apple that day. If you have two food options, and one will make you happier than the other on that day, select the happy food. Some days happy food may be french fries and other days it may be a salad. Both are fine as long as you are sticking to your plan.

Your sanity is everything, and if you are punishing yourself into eating ambiguously "clean", you are not being flexible. The beauty of this diet is that it says, "Hey, you can have your cake, and eat it too". Constantly restricting yourself isn't good for the mind.

If you read the above paragraph and said "but fruit, natural peanut butter, and salads are good and doughnuts and french fries are bad", I want you to go all the way back to page one and start from the beginning. I am encouraging you to look at food only by its macronutrient make-up while keeping the importance of micronutrients in mind. Eat healthy, but periodically enjoy your favorite foods in moderation guilt free. You are no longer bound only to chicken and veggies.

Leftover Macros

I am the administrator of a large female flexible dieting Facebook group, and we eventually had to ban the following types of questions: "*It's the end of the day and I have 5 grams of protein, 31 grams of carbs, and 18 grams of fat left, what do I eat?*"

Eat whatever the hell you want! You know what foods contain protein, carbs, and fats so use your newfound knowledge and have some fun with this game of flexible Food Tetris. Having leftover macros allows you to be creative and explore food options. The more practice you have working with "leftover macros" at the end of the day, the better you will get at flexible dieting in its entirety.

Sources & Further Reading Suggestions:

Jay R. Hoffman and Michael J. Falvo, authors. PROTEIN – WHICH IS BEST? [Internet archive] International Society of Sports Nutrition Symposium, June 18-19, 2005, Las Vegas NV, USA - Symposium - Macronutrient Utilization During Exercise: Implications For Performance And Supplementation. Journal of Sports Science and Medicine (2004) 3, 118-130. Accessed at: http://www.jssm.org/vol3/n3/2/v3n3-2pdf.pdf

The Nutrition Source. Types of Fat [Internet]. Harvard University T.H. Chan School of Public Health. Accessed 5 January 2015 at http://www.hsph.harvard.edu/nutritionsource/types-of-fat/

GROCERY GUIDE

PROTEIN:
- Chicken breast (leaner cut)
- Chicken thighs (higher fat)
- Ground turkey*
- Ground beef*
- Pork chops & other pork products
- Lamb chops & other lamb products
- Bison
- Steak (all cuts)
- Elk
- Bison
- Scallops
- Salmon (higher fat fish)
- Halibut
- Tuna steak
- Canned tuna
- Other Seafood
- Greek yogurt
- Eggs
- Egg whites
- Deli meat
- Protein Powder (all types)
- Protein Bars (all types)

*(leanness based on personal macros)

CARBS:
- All fruit
- All vegetables
- Brown or white rice
- Oats
- Potatoes and yams
- Quinoa
- Couscous
- Beans, lentils, legumes
- Popcorn
- Pasta
- Bread (all types, Ezekiel is best)
- Tortillas (corn and wheat)
- Cereal
- Most condiments/sauces: BBQ sauce, syrup, tomato sauce
- Most drinks (juices, sodas)
- Processed carbs that you find in boxes and bags (chips, crackers, etc.)

FAT:
- Coconut Oil (for cooking)
- Olive Oil (not meant to be heated)
- Other Oils
- Avocado
- Butter
- Bacon
- Nuts (all kinds)
- Nut butters (all kinds)

Once you fill up your cart or basket with the aforementioned items, you are allowed to have some fun—in moderation. All the "fun" foods tend to be made up of carbs and fat and act great as filler foods for those leftover macros you are going to encounter.

If you are an ice cream lover, head over to the freezer and grab a pint. If highly processed pastries are your thing, head over and grab those Oreos or Pop Tarts. Please just remember that the goal here is moderation and balance. When I grocery shop, I allow myself to throw two or three things in my cart that sill people would consider "bad" for me. If you buy Oreos, buy ONE pack and make it last the week. If you buy Sour Patch Kids, buy ONE bag and make it last the week. If you buy potato chips, buy ONE bag and make it last the week. So on.

Do not attempt to plan these treats into your diet ahead of time, as that's rarely how things work out. You never know when your sweet (or salt) tooth is going to kick in, thus having these things on hand keeps you prepared. Not to mention you are more accurately able to track these items with barcodes.

On the contrary, if you have a history of binging or you have been known to dust entire pints of Ben & Jerry's in one sitting, it may be best to keep these items out of reach. For right now, you know yourself better than I do, so use your best judgment in gauging your self-control.

If you choose to not indulge in store bought goods and your vice is going out to eat, keep in mind that it is a skill to track food when eating out. Eating out in moderation means less accuracy but this is the whole flexible part. If you don't have a major weight loss goal, eating out is perfectly fine when you make smart choices and still exercise some portion control. You are going to have to eyeball portions and track the best you can.

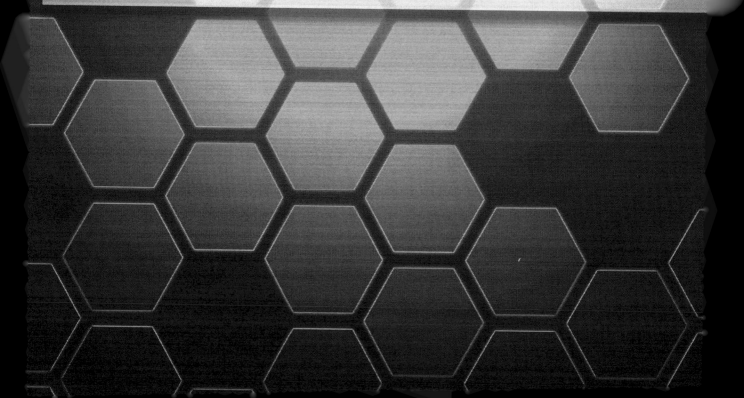

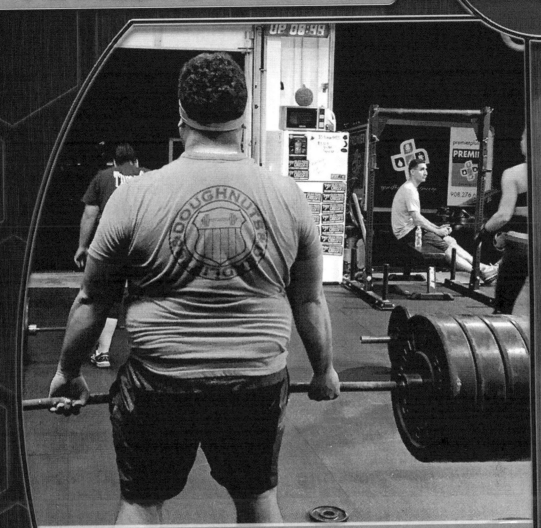

MIGUEL CARDIA
CROSSFIT

WHO ARE YOU AND WHAT DO YOU DO?

MY NAME IS MIGUEL CARDIA. I AM CROSSFIT ATHLETE & LEVEL 1 COACH. I HAVE BEEN DOING CROSSFIT FOR ABOUT 3 YEARS, AND I FELL IN LOVE WITH HELPING PEOPLE AND HOW I FELT AND WANTED TO MAKE OTHERS FEEL THE SAME WAY

WHEN DID YOU START FLEXIBLE DIETING?

I STARTED FLEXIBLE DIETING IN JULY 2013

WHAT WAS YOUR DIET LIKE BEFORE FLEXIBLE DIETING?

I STARTED WITH PALEO WHEN I STARTED CROSSFIT IN 2012 AND LOST 70LBS. AFTER HITTING A PLATEAU I WENT ON TO CARBNITE BY KIEFER. THIS CAUSED MY PERFORMANCE TO LACK IN THE GYM, ALTHOUGH MY STRENGTH WENT UP. AFTER CARBNITE, I CONTINUED TO TRY MIXING WHAT I HAVE LEARNED OVER THE YEARS UNTIL A FRIEND SHOWED ME FLEXIBLE DIETING. I BOUGHT KRISSY'S BOOK AND IMMEDIATELY FOUND INFORMATION I HAD BEEN LOOKING FOR.

WHAT HAS BEEN YOUR BIGGEST BREAKTHROUGH SINCE FLEXIBLE DIETING?

SINCE FLEXIBLE DIETING, I HAVE LEARNED TO NOT BE SCARED OF FOOD, I HAVE ALSO LEARNED HOW FOOD AND WHAT FOODS AFFECT MY PERFORMANCE DIFFERENTLY. SINCE STARTING FLEXIBLE DIETING, MY STRENGTH NUMBERS HAVE GONE UP, AND I HAVE BEEN ABLE TO CUT DOWN MY 5K ROW AND MILE RUN TIME. I HAVE REALIZED THAT I AM IN CONTROL. MOST OF ALL I AM HAPPY WITH HOW I EAT BECAUSE I CAN BE FLEXIBLE AND NOT HAVE TO FEEL GUILTY WHEN I EAT SOMETHING "BAD" (WHAT IS BAD ANYWAY?).

WHAT ARE YOUR THREE MOST IMPORTANT GUIDELINES YOU GIVE YOURSELF?

1. MAKE SURE I PLAN AHEAD ESPECIALLY WHEN I WANT TO EAT FOODS THAT MAY NOT HELP ME PERFORM AS BEST.
2. MAKE SURE I HIT MY CALORIES AND PROTEIN ABOVE ALL ELSE.
3. STAY CONSISTENT

WHAT IS THE BEST PIECE OF ADVICE YOU WISH YOU HAD WHEN STARTING FLEXIBLE DIETING THAT COULD HELP NEWBIES?

GET A SCALE! THE FIRST COUPLE WEEKS IT WILL BE AN ADJUSTMENT, BUT DON'T FEAR THE CARBS. I HAD THE MINDSET THAT I NEEDED A LOT OF FAT, AND I ACTUALLY DIDN'T. PLAN AHEAD TO MAKE SURE YOU CAN BE CONSISTENT. MOST OF ALL ENJOY YOUR FOODS AND ENJOY THEM GUILT FREE. IGNORE EVERYONE AROUND YOU WHO WILL TELL YOU YOU'RE DOING IT WRONG. FLEXIBLE DIETING REQUIRES DISCIPLINE, AND IS NOT A FREE FOR ALL, BUT YOU WILL BE ABLE TO DO IT FOR LIFE AND BE MUCH HAPPIER.

13. Rest Day Macros

If you train hard, you are probably wondering what the hell to do with your nutrition on a rest day. If your multiplier was relatively high, you calculated how many calories you need to sustain your intense training, so what do you do on days with minimal or no activity? When you are resting from training you are giving your body an opportunity to recover . Your muscles repair themselves the days following vigorous training and by now you are aware that they do this with carbohydrates and amino acids from protein, so a rest day should never be a deprivation day. There are a few different ways to treat rest day nutrition. I don't necessarily think that there is a definitive right or wrong way because you need to find what best suits you, which means your goals are going to be the deciding factor. If you are trying to lose weight, your rest day is going to be treated differently than someone who has an upcoming weightlifting meet.

If flexible dieting is new to you and you are having trouble hitting one set of numbers, I don't suggest incorporating a second set of numbers. In the past, I have made clients prove that they can successfully and consistently hit one set of numbers for a few weeks before I allow them to throw another set into the mix. The most important factor is going to be doing what is reasonable for you despite what you see everyone doing (or say they are doing) on social media.

The Two Schools of Thought

There are two ways to look at a rest day: from a mental standpoint and from a physical standpoint. Depending on your training and your past relationship with food, one will sound more appealing than the other.

Mental Rest Day: Some people benefit from a day off of paying attention to what foods they are consuming at what times. If you are easily stressed out by nutrition, a mental rest day should be in order. If you are going to take this route, don't worry about tracking and weighing food on your rest day. Now don't get too excited because a rest day is by no means a "free" day. This isn't a hall pass from your diet. You are still required to make healthy decisions and not overindulge, but you can take a mental break from any monotonous tracking you may be doing. Simply put, you are resting your mind from having to think about nutrition.

Physical Rest Day: If you are a competitive athlete, are training for something in particular, or your multiplier was above a 13, you likely look at your scheduled rest days from a more physical point of view. A rest day is a break from your strenuous training program where you are giving your body a chance to relax. If you have "active recovery" days where you aren't putting yourself through hell and instead you mobilize, do skill work, or light activity, you can count that as a rest day. Since your rest days lack the intensity that your training days have, typically fewer calories and carbs are needed.

If You Are Eating At A Deficit

If you are already on a deficit, dropping your calories slightly on rest days is probably unnecessary, especially if you are seeing results by consistently hitting the same numbers each day. There is no reason to put yourself at a further deficit if you are making progress as this takes us back to the profound "Don't Fix It If It's Not Broken" philosophy.

If you plateau, you may opt to lower calories only on rest days in order to put yourself at a further deficit without lowering calories on training days when you will need them.

If You Are Eating At Maintenance

If your multiplier was higher on the scale, you are likely eating at a fairly high maintenance and those extra calories, specifically carbs, are not needed on your rest days. In this case, it is completely acceptable (and probably smart) to lower them on days you're not partaking in rigorous training.

Drop your carbs by 20-25% on your rest days, but leave protein and fat the same. For example, if you are consuming 200g carbs a day, you can drop to 150-160g on rest days. Another common method is to reduce your carbs to a 1:1 ratio with protein. Both these options have proven to be effective in many different athletes. Do what is easiest for you.

If You Are Eating At A Surplus

Yet again, I am going to tell you to just EAT. There isn't really any reason to alter carbs on rest days. I know some people who have been eating at a surplus for a long time and they choose to take a mental rest from time to time, which is completely fine.

If you have an exceptionally high carb intake, and you don't want to consume it all on a rest day, you can follow the guideline for maintenance, which is to lower by 20-25%.

14. Refeed Days

A refeed day is a scheduled high carb day, and is crucial if you've been on a caloric deficit for a long period of time. The purpose of a refeed is to replenish your glycogen stores and raise leptin levels. Leptin may be a new term for some of you, or you may have heard it but never understood its function. Leptin is commonly referred to as the "mother of all fat burning hormones". Leptin is a hormone in our bodies that is essentially a metabolism-controller and hunger-regulator, and its primary job is to tell the brain that we are full after a meal. However, after prolonged periods of running a caloric deficit, leptin levels can become so low that the message never makes it to the brain. Our brains actually realize that leptin is low and assume that we are not properly fueled, thus causing hunger pangs and cravings. Refeeds will raise leptin levels, regulate metabolism and decrease cravings. Think of a "refeed" as a "reboot" for your metabolism.

To repeat what I said in the last chapter, if you are having a difficult time being consistent with one set of numbers, please refrain from adding in rest days and refeed days until you get the hang of all this. Juggling three sets numbers is something that takes time to learn how to do.

A Refeed Day IS NOT a "Cheat Day"

Refeeding is not binge eating on whatever you please; it is planned and calculated. While you are increasing carbohydrates on a refeed day, your other macros will remain the same. Sure, you may use this day to indulge a little bit, but don't get too excited because it's only carbs that will increase and not your fat. Why is it important that your refeed only consist of an increase in carbs? Because, carbohydrates are converted to glucose, and leptin responds directly to glucose metabolism.

Do not justify having a case of "the fuckits" by calling it a refeed.

Who Needs It

In order to determine whether you need a refeed or not you need to think about a few things. Anyone with a lower body fat percentage (≤10% for men, and ≤15% for women) is going to need at least one refeed a week. If you are on a particularly long cut (12-16 weeks) you will most likely want to incorporate 2 refeeds a week. If you have only been on a deficit for a few weeks, you will probably not need a refeed quite yet, especially if you are seeing results. I recommend implementing a refeed day no sooner than 4 weeks into your cut, and that is only if you have plateaued. I think you know by now that losing weight is a relatively simple process that gets over-complicated by an industry that profits on misinformation. A refeed is necessary per se, and the benefits have been thoroughly discussed. It is important to remember to not do anything that is going to drive you insane or complicate the process. If you are already confused by a refeed day, you may want to do some further research and forego implementing one until you feel comfortable and better understand the reasoning.

If you are eating at maintenance, you most likely don't need to refeed.

Some athletes (myself included) like to increase carbs on their most demanding training days, but we will talk about that in the following chapter as that's a form of carb cycling and does not necessarily constitute a refeed.

If you are eating at a surplus, you probably feel like every day is a refeed day and you won't need to worry about incorporating one. How fun is bulking? I know, right?

How To Configure It

When planning a refeed, you are going to increase the amount of carbohydrates that you consume by at least 50% (some people go up to 100%) of your daily intake. For example, if you are consuming 150 grams of carbs a day on a cut, increase by 75 grams on refeed day to total 225 grams. If you want to do further research on configuring and optimizing refeed days, there is a lot of information out there to help you do so.

When To Take It

The timing of your refeed day is important as well, and it should definitely be planned. First of all, never plan your refeed on the day before a rest day.

Beyond this, there are some discrepancies and conflicting arguments by professionals about the optimal time to incorporate a refeed. An athlete trying to cut weight for a meet will be treated differently than someone on a weight loss journey.

Athletes: As you will see in the next chapter, carb cycling is simply manipulating carb intake based around training volume and intensity. For an athlete, refeed day (or days) should be introduced on max effort training days.

Weight loss: If you hit a plateau or are experiencing severe cravings, a refeed day will most likely benefit you. Try refeeding the day prior to your most intense training day (it will usually be a lower body day). Although it is less common, some people choose to refeed on their off days, which is an excellent way to allow your muscles to recover. If you choose to do this, make sure that you have a very intense training day the following day.

When it comes to refeeds, there is no equation to determine either the perfect amount of carbs, or the optimal day on which to do so. You can enlist a coach to help you optimize your refeed days, or you can experiment with some trial and error on your own to see what feels best both mentally and physically. One thing I do want you to try and avoid is "earning" your refeed day through exercise. Just stick to your training program and know that a refeed is well deserved by those who adhere to their plan.

By throwing the above mentioned "refeed" and "rest" days into your plan, you are essentially carb cycling. Carb cycling is exactly what it implies: cycling your carbs between low, moderate, and high days. The goal is to manipulate them in such a way that it improves performance and body composition. People have seen great aesthetic results with carb cycling when done right through the help of a knowledgeable coach. People have seen greater performance results by increasing carbs on difficult training days for obvious reasons (increased glycogen).

15. Carb Cycling For Athletes

Increasing carbs on demanding, heavy training days is a surefire way to enhance your training. The reason this isn't necessarily a "refeed" is because you are not consuming more carbs for the sake of leptin, but rather for fuel, and to hopefully improve the quality of your performance. You will be using the extra amount you take in.

If you are trying to lose weight, or have strictly aesthetic goals, I do think that carb cycling is somewhat unnecessary for a few reasons:

1. Consistency purposes. The entire goal with this is to create consistency by allowing some flexibility. When you start attempting to hit three sets of numbers each week, you are steering away from your foundation. Furthermore, since you will be all over the map with numbers, it will be difficult to pinpoint why you aren't losing weight should weight loss start to plateau. Which numbers do you tweak? Who knows.

2. It all balances out by the end of the week. If you consume 20% more carbs two days a week and 20% less carbs two days a week, you'd be eating exactly what you originally would have had you just stuck to the initial caloric goal. This is why carb cycling works for performance, but isn't a huge asset for weight loss.

3. If you are on a cut and you're not a competitive athlete, your training probably isn't at a level that requires a carb influx.

If you are on a deficit in order to lose weight, performance is clearly a secondary goal and sticking to the same numbers daily along with refeeds when needed is best. If you are an athlete who is looking to become a better athlete, carb cycling is an excellent tool that you should utilize once you have a firm grasp on flexible dieting.

How It's Done

Like rest days, manipulate carbs by 20-25%. The increase should obviously come before and after your training to top off and replenish your glycogen stores. My athletes tend to notice a quicker recovery rate when more carbs are introduced post workout which is perfect since you are implementing this on your max effort days. Fat gain won't take place since training volume and intensity are increased.

It shouldn't be too difficult to decide which day (or days) are your most demanding. If you are a competitive athlete, there are surely days where you train 2 or 3 times, or have a 4-5 hour session, in which case liquid carbs can be consumed during training. Consider Gatorade® and Vitargo® as options here.

16. Reverse Dieting

Dr. Norton has pioneered the practice of Reverse Dieting over the last few years, and it is a very interesting and compelling subject. Reverse dieting is for anyone looking to maximize their metabolic capacity.

"Reverse dieting is a form of positive metabolic adaptation in which the body responds in a favorable manner to increased food intake. This is achieved via a controlled diet of steadily increasing macronutrient intake and is designed to prime you metabolically without gaining excess body fat." -Sohee Lee

If you have been dieting too hard for too long, you're going to eventually hit a wall, which is not easy to recover from. Example time:

Let's say someone is 200 pounds and wants to lose 50 pounds. Said person immediately slashes their calories and consumes 1200 calories a day for 7 months and loses that 50 pounds despite feeling tired and hungry for over half a year. What now? Rather than reintroducing 500 calories right away, which could potentially put all that weight back on very quickly, the idea is to gradually and subtly increase calories over the course of several weeks (or possibly months depending on the situation) to get back to good standing. "Good standing" meaning sanity being restored, or getting to a place where weight loss can continue in a healthy manner that doesn't involve drastic calorie restriction.

With Reverse Dieting, you gradually introduce carbs and fat on a weekly or bi-weekly basis until your baseline is high and healthy enough to sustain your desired lifestyle. How do you do this? By increasing carbs and fats by roughly 10% each week.

There is much more to it than simply "increasing carbs and fat by 10% each week" due to the fact that each person is a unique case and should be treated as such. It takes a lot of consistency and body awareness to reverse diet successfully. Not to mention the psychological component that goes hand in hand with it.

Luckily the experts, Norton and Lee, wrote a book on this that can better assist you if you're curious to explore Reverse Dieting further. If you have been chronically under eating and having a scoop of ice cream causes you to gain a pound, it's safe to say reading their book is worth your time and money.

"The truth is, there is no clinical definition for metabolic adaptation. As a relatively new concept, there have unfortunately been no scientific studies done on the topic to date. But first, let's clear the air. Originally coined by Scott Abel, the term metabolic damage describes a phenomenon in which the body refuses to shed fat despite what would typically be considered dieting calories and activity levels. Conversely, the body may also experience fat gain in excess of what is predicted by caloric intake and activity level. In this book, we prefer to utilize the

more descriptive term metabolic adaptation. Note that the two terms can typically be used interchangeably. But even so, this definition doesn't quite suffice, as there are numerous caveats. For one, after a long stint of low calorie dieting, weight gain is normal and expected. This is often observed in bodybuilding competitors who, after a long prep season, may overeat or even binge eat. When this happens, the competitor is said to be going through a rebound, which is distinct from metabolic damage because the individual is putting him or herself into a caloric surplus, albeit unintentionally." - Sohee Lee & Dr. Layne Norton, *Reverse Dieting.*

Beyond reverse dieting back from extreme deprivation, you can use it on a perfectly healthy metabolism as well. Reverse dieting from maintaining at 2200 calories up to 2800 calories is what allowed me to cut weight on a 2300-2400 calorie diet. I've known powerlifters who have slowly reverse dieted up to 4000 calories, which allowed them to cut an insane amount of weight on 3000 calories. Cutting on this many calories tends to prevent strength and performance loss. How's that sound? Pretty good, I think.

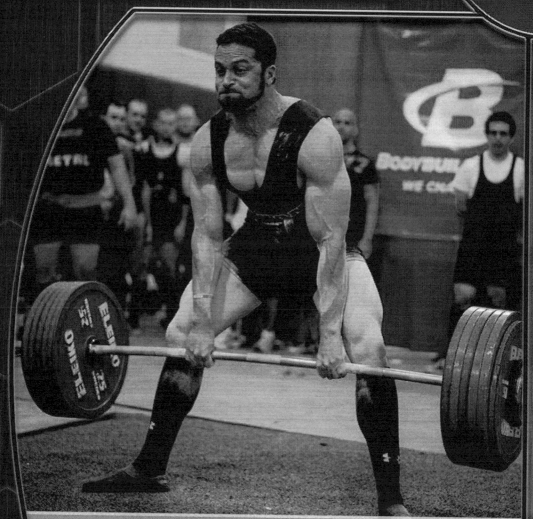

DR. LAYNE NORTON

BODYBUILDING/POWERLIFTING

WWW.BIOLAYNE.COM
YOUTUBE: WWW.YOUTUBE.COM/BIOLAYNE
FACEBOOK: WWW.FACEBOOK.COM/LAYNENORTON
TWITTER: WWW.TWITTER.COM/BIOLAYNE
INSTAGRAM: WWW.INSTAGRAM.COM/BIOLAYNE

DR. LAYNE NORTON

EVEN THOUGH YOU NEED NO INTRODUCTION, GO AHEAD AND TELL US WHO YOU ARE AND WHAT YOU DO.

BASICALLY I'M A SCIENCE GEEK WHO ALSO LIKES TO LIFT HEAVY SHIT AND LOOK GOOD. I DID MY BS IN BIOCHEMISTRY AND MY PHD IN NUTRITIONAL SCIENCES. I HAVE PRO STATUS IN NATURAL BODYBUILDING AND POWERLIFTING. I WON 2014 USAPL RAW NATIONALS TO QUALIFY FOR 2015 IPF WORLDS.

WHEN DID YOU START COMPETITIVE POWERLIFTING AND HOW BIG OF A ROLE WOULD YOU SAY FLEXIBLE DIETING HAS PLAYED IN YOUR STRENGTH AND PERFORMANCE?

I STARTED IN 2008 AFTER STRUGGLING WITH STAYING MOTIVATED DURING MY BODYBUILDING OFFSEASON. I HAD TROUBLE ENJOYING MY TRAINING WHEN I WASN'T GETTING READY FOR A SHOW, POWERLIFTING WAS A NICE OUTLET TO GIVE ME CONCRETE GOALS TO MAKE PROGRESS AND ENJOY TRAINING OTHER THAN TO JUST 'GAIN MUSCLE' WHICH IS SUCH A SLOW PROCESS MOST TIMES YOU DON'T EVEN KNOW IF YOU ARE MAKING PROGRESS. BUT I KNOW IF I'M SQUATTING MORE WEIGHT THAN I WAS A MONTH AGO AND EASIER TO SEE THAT TANGIBLE PROGRESS. FLEXIBLE DIETING HAS BEEN EXTREMELY HELPFUL TO KEEP ME CONSISTENT DAY IN AND DAY OUT, WEEK IN AND WEEK OUT, YEAR IN AND YEAR OUT. WHILE OTHER GUYS ARE HAVING TO CUT 10-20 LBS TO MAKE WEIGH INS BECAUSE THEY SAY 'SCREW IT' WHEN THEY AREN'T COMPETING, I PRETTY MUCH MAINTAIN AND TRAIN AT MY COMPETITION WEIGHT ALL YEAR ROUND, WHICH FOR ME IS PRETTY DARN LEAN, BECAUSE IT IS A LIFESTYLE FOR ME.

WHAT BENEFITS DO COMPETITIVE STRENGTH ATHLETES TEND TO SEE ONCE ADOPTING FLEXIBLE DIETING THAT THEY MAY HAVE BEEN MISSING PRIOR TO FAMILIARIZING THEMSELVES WITH OPTIMIZING MACRONUTRIENT INTAKE?

WHEN YOU UNDERSTAND WHAT YOUR PROTEIN, CARB, FAT INTAKE IS, IT TAKES THE GUESSWORK OUT OF THINGS. YOU KNOW WHAT YOU GAIN ON, KNOW WHAT YOU MAINTAIN ON, AND YOU KNOW WHAT YOU LOSE ON. THERE IS VERY LITTLE GUESS WORK. FURTHER, BECAUSE THERE ARE NO DIETARY RESTRICTIONS OTHER THAN HITTING YOUR MACRONUTRIENT INTAKE, IT IS FAR EASIER FOR PEOPLE TO BE CONSISTENT WITH IT RATHER THAN PUTTING ON 20-30-40-50 LBS IN BETWEEN MEETS THEN HAVING TO CRASH DIET TO LOSE IT.

YOU ARE EXTREMELY WELL KNOWN IN THE AESTHETICS SIDE OF THIS BUSINESS. HOW DOES FLEXIBLE DIETING DIFFER FOR PERFORMANCE ATHLETES AND AESTHETIC ATHLETES?

NOT MUCH AT ALL. WHAT MAINTAINS MUSCLE BEST WILL MAINTAIN STRENGTH BEST DURING DIETING. SO THE APPROACH IS LARGELY THE SAME, THOUGH THE ABSOLUTE TARGET OUTCOMES ARE A BIT DIFFERENT.

WHAT WOULD YOU SAY ARE THE THREE MOST IMPORTANT GENERAL GUIDELINES

STRENGTH AND PERFORMANCE ATHLETES SHOULD FOLLOW WHEN IT COMES TO NUTRITION?

- CONSISTENCY IS KEY! NO MATTER WHAT YOU DO, MAKE IT A LIFESTYLE. OTHERWISE YOU WILL BE RIDING THE ROLLER COASTER OF GAINING & LOSING WEIGHT, GAINING AND LOSING WEIGHT. AND IF YOU DO IT WRONG, EACH TIME IT WILL GET HARDER AND HARD TO LOSE IT.

- EATING SUFFICIENT PROTEIN, BUT NOT EXCESSIVE. 1G/LB IS MORE THAN ENOUGH FOR OPTIMAL MUSCLE MASS AND STRENGTH. IF YOU WANT TO EAT MORE BECAUSE YOU LIKE PROTEIN, FINE BUT IT'S NOT GIVING YOU BETTER RESULTS FOR STRENGTH AND EATING TOO MUCH IS PROBABLY COUNTER PRODUCTIVE.

- STOP CRASH DIETING FOR MEETS. I REMEMBER A POWERLIFTER AT MY GYM WITH A TOP SQUAT OF 650. HE WANTED TO COMPETE AT 198 AND WAS SITTING ABOUT 230 A MONTH OUT. NO PROBLEM HE SAID, HE'D JUST DROP IT IN A MONTH. WELL HE BOMBED OUT OF HIS MEET, DIDN'T EVEN HIT HIS OPENER. YOU SIMPLY CANNOT LET YOURSELF GET THAT FAR OUT OF WHAT WEIGHT YOU COMPETE AT AND EXPECT TO PERFORM OPTIMALLY.

WE WERE ALL NEW TO THIS AT SOME POINT (INCLUDING YOU, DOC). WHAT IS THE SINGLE BEST PIECE OF ADVICE YOU WISH YOU HAD WHEN FIRST STARTING FLEXIBLE DIETING AND POWERLIFTING THAT COULD HELP NEWBIES?

BE PATIENT. NO ONE SQUATS 600 LBS OVERNIGHT. IF YOU WANT TO BECOME GREAT AT SOMETHING IT WILL TAKE MOST PEOPLE A DECADE... MINIMUM. YOU WILL HAVE TO PUT IN TENS OF THOUSANDS OF HOURS TRAINING. MOST OF THE BEST POWERLIFTERS WENT THROUGH THE SAME TRIALS AND TRIBULATIONS AS THE REST OF US... THE DIFFERENCE IS THAT THEY KEPT GRINDING THROUGH WHEN EVERYONE ELSE GAVE UP AND QUIT. IF YOU QUIT, OR GO THROUGH PHASES OF LOW MOTIVATION WHERE YOU STOP, IT JUST SETS YOU BACK FURTHER. UNDERSTAND THAT MOTIVATION WILL COME AND GO AND MANY TIMES YOU WILL HAVE TO GRIND WHEN YOU DON'T FEEL LIKE TRACKING SOMETHING OR EVEN LOOKING AT A BARBELL.

MANY PEOPLE RECENTLY SAW ME DROP A SIGNIFICANT AMOUNT OF WEIGHT WHILE PREPPING TO COMPETE WITH NO LOSS OF STRENGTH. DO YOU THINK CUTTING WEIGHT WHILE GAINING (OR EVEN MAINTAINING) STRENGTH IS A PSYCHOLOGICAL PROCESS, OR IS IT ATTRIBUTED TO PROPER NUTRITION AND PROGRAMMING?

IT'S BOTH. I SEE MANY PEOPLE RESIGN THEMSELVES TO LOSING STRENGTH WHEN CUTTING. NEWSFLASH, IF YOU BELIEVE YOU WILL LOSE STRENGTH... YOU WILL LOSE STRENGTH. I DROPPED FROM 220 TO 205 AND ADDED 30 LBS TO MY SQUAT, 5 LBS TO MY BENCH, AND 20 LBS TO MY DEADLIFT, BUT I DID IT OVER THE COURSE OF 9 MONTHS AND WAS METICULOUS AND CONSISTENT.

17. Eating Out

There are two kinds of "going out to eat". The kind you do out of convenience, and the kind you do to spend time with people you care about and make memories. It is important to differentiate the two. If you are eating out to enjoy your time with another human being, order what will make you happy and make the experience a memorable one. You don't have to order a dry chicken breast with steamed broccoli. On the other hand, if you are eating out because it is convenient, you should make a solid effort to order something relatively healthy that can be accounted for.

Remember, this lifestyle is a *choice*. You can easily stay on track without sacrificing your social life or alienating yourself because you've chosen to be on a "diet". There's no reason why food should come between you and your friends, or between you and your goals for that matter. There is always a healthier or better option on the menu; it's about choosing correctly and making sure you stick to your plan.

Adhering to Macros When Eating Out

Eating out isn't a difficult task when it comes to flexible dieting. I want to stress that this is supposed to be a lifestyle. Ultimately, the objective is to find something that allows you to meet your health and fitness goals, but still allows you to live your life. You should not have to sacrifice any sort of social life in order to achieve your goals. You do not want to be the person who brings their Tupperware meals or their food scale to a restaurant.

__Learn portion sizes__: If you're in the habit of weighing your food, which you damn well better be if you're tracking properly, then you should pay attention to the visual size of your portions. Get familiar with what 6 ounces of chicken breast looks like. When you go out to eat you can order chicken and be able to estimate the proper amount of protein you're consuming. Furthermore, it's okay to ask questions. You typically won't see meat listed by the ounce on a menu unless you're ordering a steak, but if you really need to know and you're not able to eyeball it, ask your server. Chances are the restaurant staff is familiar with portions sizes.

__Use the app__: When I say that MFP has an impressive food database, I am not over-exaggerating. Almost every chain restaurant is in MFP, from In-N-Out and Chipotle to Smith & Wollensky's and Ruth's Chris. It is very easy to accurately track as most restaurants disclose nutritional information in MFP, or on their websites.

__Plan ahead__: Look at the menu ahead of time and make a plan. If you know you are meeting a friend for lunch in the next few days, go online and look at the menu. Enter what you plan to eat (this takes us back to Chapter Ten), record the macros, and make adjustments, if necessary. Above all, stick to your plan.

__If there's no nutritional info available__: When ordering, choose your protein source first and build your meal from there. Fish or chicken will usually be your leanest options, steak will have a good amount of fat in it and it's harder to guesstimate the nutritional value since every cut of meat will be differently marbled and vary in its fat content. Once you've decided on your protein, you can choose your carb and fat sources. Ask for substitutions if it will put your mind at ease. Don't be afraid to ask how something is prepared. You can always ask to have your food cooked with no seasonings, no butter, and no oil. Don't go crazy and order something with 17 ingredients as that gets tough to track if it's not inventoried in MFP. Be careful with salads, which are ordinarily a safe option, unless they are drowning in dressing and have all kinds of sneaky toppings.

If you are going somewhere worth starving for, another option would be to save up most of your macros for that meal. Eat less throughout the day so that you'll have more leftover macros to work with when you go out. For example, if you know you're planning on going to your favorite pizza joint for dinner, stick to meals consisting of mostly protein for breakfast and lunch. This way you'll have ample carbs and fat left for your pizza. Do not do this on a regular basis because then we are venturing into "IIFYM" territory, and I want your insides to look just as good as your outsides.

Not Adhering To Macros When Eating Out

Provided you are more than 4 weeks out from competing in bodybuilding, you can get away with being a little more flexible when the occasion calls for it. Weddings, graduations, promotions, birthdays, anniversaries, and other important events deserve to be celebrated with zero nutritional stress. **Treat yo'self**. Don't let feelings of food guilt ruin a special night with people you love.

There is a third kind of eating out that I wanted to save until the very end of this chapter, the kind where you travel hours out of your way to try a doughnut burger. That kind deserves no fucks. Dig in.

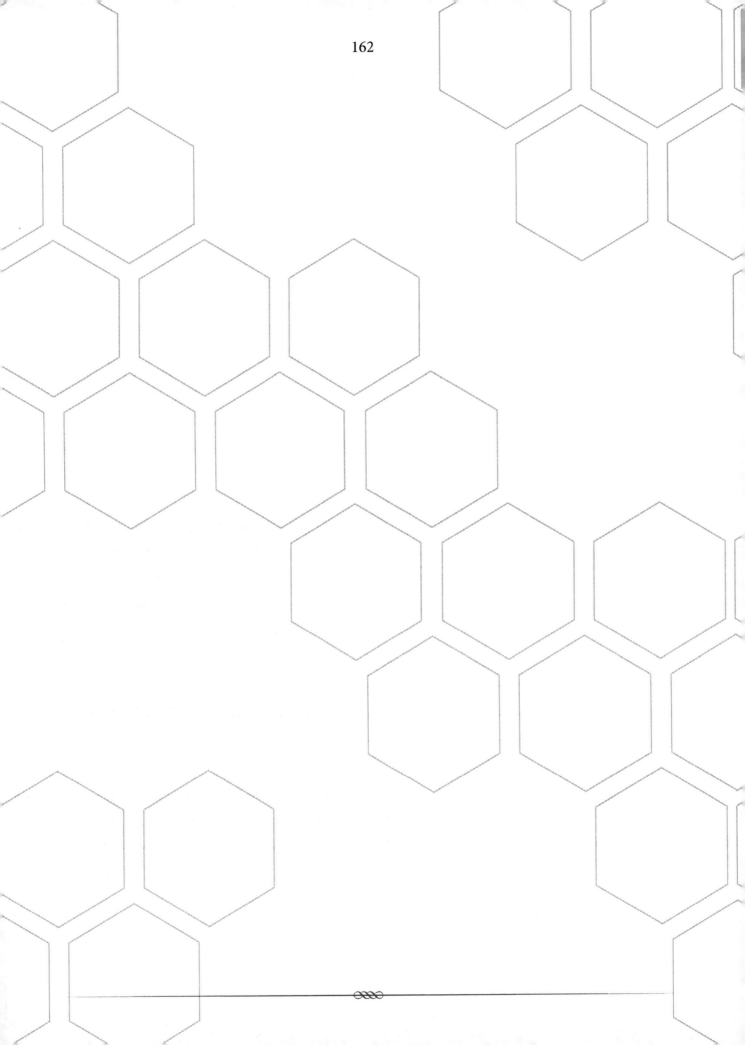

18. Supplementation

If you know anything about me, you know my stance on supplements. I'm generally not a fan, nor do I promote the use of many supplements. I have personal issues with the supplement companies' advertising and marketing agendas. I think they give the general population false hope by suggesting that a fitness model's body can be achieved with creatine, pre-workout powders, and fat burners.

Before you supplement your diet, your diet should be worth supplementing. If you are incapable of consistently hitting the same number of calories for a few weeks, supplementation should probably be the last thing on your mind when it comes to nutrition. Fat burners aren't going to do shit if you are eating above maintenance. From an aesthetic perspective, I think adhering to what is outlined in this book will yield the results you're looking for, and save you the money you would have otherwise wasted on ineffective and superfluous supplements.

I do understand that some people have persistent vitamin and mineral deficiencies for an array of reasons, in which case a vitamin supplement would be recommended. However, if you are deficient because you eat like an asshole, you can fix that problems sans pills. Don't take a multivitamin for the sake of taking one. Know why you are taking one.

My advice? Keep it simple. And only support brands who represent the industry well and send a positive message.

Caffeine: This is a no brainer, we all love it. I prefer a good cup of coffee over pre-workout supplements and thermogenics. Caffeine is a widely known stimulant which means it can suppress appetite, improve mood, and increase energy. Caffeine is well researched and safe, which is not a claim that thermogenics can boast. My preferred caffeine source is Caveman Coffee.

Protein: As we've already covered, there is a time and a place for protein supplementation. The great thing about protein powder is its exceptionally high bioavailability. A second perk is that the price per serving is far more affordable than meat. The vast number of types and brands available on the market can be overwhelming, but I have some good news for you: most of it comes from the same place and it's almost all the same shit aside from flavor alterations. I personally choose high quality and grass-fed whey or vegan protein from Gnarly Nutrition, which is a company that delivers a positive message along with a superior, great tasting product.

BCAAs: Branched chain amino acids are essential nutrients and another awesome tool for optimizing muscle protein synthesis (particularly leucine). We have repeatedly discussed the importance of amino acids throughout the book and supplementing your diet with them can be beneficial to prevent muscle breakdown, especially while eating at a deficit. Like protein powder, the choices are overwhelming. Also, like protein powder, it's all the same shit. Again, I choose Gnarly because I like the company and what it promotes.

Supplements for Athletic Performance

There are many supplements shown to aid in the performance and recovery of athletes, and it's a subject matter that could fill an entire book of its own. It's an area where I am admittedly not as well-versed, but am presently studying more intently (that's a hint for something I am currently working on). Once you nail down flexible dieting, I urge you to explore the Journal of The International Society of Sports Nutrition if performance supplementation is something that interests you.

19. Conclusion

Upon finishing this book, the following sentence should stick with you: Your body doesn't make the same distinctions between foods that your mind does.

If nutrition were as simple as "eat less and lose fat, eat more and gain muscle", every single one of us would have a phenomenal physique. Eating habits are extremely rooted in our emotions and psychology, which means that our behavioral patterns must necessarily change to develop a healthier relationship with food. Get your mind right, then get your diet right. Masking emotional issues with single digit body fat won't fix them.

My job as a nutrition professional is not to beat what is and is not healthy into your head. It is not my job to give you a list of foods that are "good for you" along with a list of foods that are "off limits". I am not the food police. I like cheeseburgers and doughnuts, but I also really like salmon and asparagus. Have some pizza or ice cream, but not every single day. I believe in balance over everything, as that is an indicator of true health. My job as a nutrition professional is to educate you on how to take care of yourself and fuel your life.

Do not use fitness to earn your food or to counteract poor eating behavior, instead, use it to get strong. Lift weights, train hard, and love every second of it.

You now have an effective philosophy for determining your own nutrition that you will have at your disposal for the rest of your life. You know how to eat flexibly, how to accurately track your macros, and how to alter your eating to support your goals. It is up to you to make the lifestyle change and put this information into action. All that is required of you is consistency, patience, and of course, some flexibility.

Yours in doughnut & deadlifts,
Krissy Mae Cagney

MACRO CHEAT SHEET

2. HOW MUCH DO YOU WORK OUT?

×11=SEDENTARY
×12=LESS THAN 5 HRS/WK
×13=5-10 HRS/WK
×14=10-15 HRS/WK
×15=15-20 HRS/WK
×16=20+ HRS/WK
*ADD 0.5 TO YOUR NUMBER
IF YOU HAVE AN ACTIVE JOB

1. WHAT DO YOU WEIGH?

3. YOU NEED THIS MANY CALORIES.

DETERMINE YOUR CALORIES
(MAINTENANCE CALORIES)

1. YOUR WEIGHT (IN LBS):_____

×

2. LIFESTYLE MULTIPLIER:_____

=

3. DAILY CALORIC NEEDS:_____

WHAT IS YOUR GOAL?

CUTTING

- START AT MAINTENANCE THEN SUBTRACT 100-1000KCAL
- THE SIZE OF YOUR DEFICIT DEPENDS ON YOUR CURRENT LEVEL OF LEANNESS
- THE LEANER YOU ARE, THE SMALLER THE DEFICIT NEEDS TO BE

MAINTENANCE-DEFICIT

_____ - _____ = _____ =KCAL FOR YOUR CUT

MAINTENANCE

EAT AT MAINTENANCE FOR:
- PERFORMANCE AND
- BODY RECOMPOSITION

BULKING

- START WITH MAINTENANCE THEN ADD 500-1000KCAL
- IF YOU WANT A SLOW GAIN, STAY AT THE LOWER END. IF YOU WANT BIG GAINS, GO NUTS
- EXPECT A SMALL AMOUNT OF FAT GAIN

MAINTENANCE + SURPLUS

_____ + _____ = _____ =KCAL FOR YOUR BULK

1 G PER LB (BETWEEN CURRENT BODYWEIGHT & LEAN BODY MASS)
OR
2 G PER KG OF BODYWEIGHT

_____ ×4=KCALS FROM PROTEIN

0.4-0.5 G PER LB OF BODYWEIGHT
OR
1 G PER KG OF BODYWEIGHT

_____ ×9=KCALS FROM FAT

NOW FIND YOUR MACROS

CARBS MAKE UP THE REMAINDER OF YOUR CALORIC TOTAL. ADD CALORIES FROM FAT AND PROTEIN THEN SUBTRACT THAT FROM TOTAL CALORIES.

THIS IS YOUR KCAL FROM CARBS. DIVIDE BY 4

_____ = _____ THIS IS HOW MANY G OF CARBS.

- CREATE MEAL APPROACHES THAT WORK FOR YOU AND YOUR LIFESTYLE, YOUR SCHEDULE, YOUR PREFERENCES
- HITTING YOUR PROTEIN IS MOST IMPORTANT. THERE CAN BE WIGGLE ROOM AMONGST FATS AND CARBS AS LONG AS PROTEIN AND TOTAL CALORIES ARE BEING MET
- TWEAK YOUR CARBS AND FAT IF YOU ARE CONSISTENTLY ABOVE ON ONE AND BELOW ON ANOTHER
- BE CONSISTENT FOR TWO WEEKS IN ORDER TO GAUGE HOW ACCURATE YOUR CALCULATIONS ARE. TWEAK ACCORDINGLY, IF NECESSARY

- DON'T DICK AROUND AND THEN THINK THE NUMBERS YOU AREN'T HITTING DON'T WORK
- YOU CAN'T CHEAT THE PROCESS
- IF ON A CUT, DOING TOO BIG OF A CUT WON'T ACCELERATE YOUR PROGRESS
- WEIGH YOURSELF, BUT NOT EVERY DAY. IF YOUR SCALE DOESN'T MOVE FOR TWO WEEKS, YOU ARE AT BASELINE. CUT, BULK, MAINTAIN AS YOU NEED
- RECALCULATE EVERY 6 WEEKS OR 10-15 POUNDS
- EAT. LIFT. LIVE.

THESE ARE YOUR MACROS